Also by Inge Trachtenberg:
An Arranged Marriage
So Slow the Dawning

My Daughter My Son

by Inge Trachtenberg

WITH CONTRIBUTIONS BY
SUSAN TRACHTENBERG

SUMMIT BOOKS
NEW YORK

PUBLISHED BY SUMMIT BOOKS
A SIMON & SCHUSTER DIVISION OF GULF & WESTERN CORPORATION
SIMON & SCHUSTER BUILDING
ROCKEFELLER CENTER
1230 AVENUE OF THE AMERICAS
NEW YORK, NEW YORK 10020

DESIGNED BY EVE METZ
MANUFACTURED IN THE UNITED STATES OF AMERICA

1 2 3 4 5 6 7 8 9 10

LIBRARY OF CONGRESS CATALOGING IN PUBLICATION DATA
TRACHTENBERG, INGE.
    MY DAUGHTER, MY SON.
    BIBLIOGRAPHY: P.
    1. ULCERATIVE COLITIS IN CHILDREN—BIOGRAPHY.
2. ILEOSTOMY—BIOGRAPHY. 3. TRACHTENBERG,
SUSAN. I. TRACHTENBERG, SUSAN, JOINT AUTHOR.
II. TITLE.
RJ456.C74T72   362.1'9'75540926   78–16962
ISBN 0–671–40043–6

Because there are no words needed between us, just:
to Mike

Prologue

This is a true account; true as seen through my eyes; felt and sifted and interpreted by my perceptions. Then why have I chosen to give ficticious names to my children, my husband, the doctors, the nurses and myself? Was it to disguise our identities? To give us privacy? Why the masquerade?

I have no real answer to this question. Except, perhaps, to explain that I need a device while telling this story, a device that will lend a little distance, a haziness, an illusion of separateness. Maybe, if I had waited to write this book, if I were to write it two years hence, time would give me this perspective much more naturally. But since I am writing it now, writing it while we are still living it, writing it before it is ended, I need a little help. And beg the reader's indulgence. . . .

CHAPTER 1

JUNE 3, 1965
The Day
7 A.M.

Still under wraps of sleeping veils
awareness rushes back, assails,
and it is morning of the day
and I must wake and start to pray.

No more, no more the speculation . . .
end of the road, of hesitation;
this is the morning of the day
I am awake and I must pray.

1 P.M.

All the prayers ended, the tears shed
there is this nothingness, this waiting,
this staring at his empty bed,
my mind is blank, a barren thing.

I closed the heavy iron gate
upon my colored images . . .
I blocked out red, the tint of hate,
and I breathe shallow and feel less.

MARCH 4, 1977

The Day

Only now it is her bed, not his, and I am no longer rhyming. Or really praying either, though, of course, I catch myself clutching my hands, saying inside: God, please . . . But it only makes me feel angry and ashamed. Yet, amazingly, the poem still works almost perfectly, its emotional quality and even the images. But then, why not? Here we are again: the same hospital, the same terror, and Mark and I. Mark and I, almost twelve years older than we were at the time of Samson's surgery. So is he, of course; Sam sits with us now in Rachel's hospital room, having taken the day off from law school, going through whatever his particular agony is in reliving this as an adult. Certainly he has been the one most helpful to Rachel these last few days and this morning at six before they wheeled her off.

So we sit and stare at her empty bed and talk about the way everything is better now—progress. For instance, that they did not insert the various tubes and catheters while Rachel was still awake, and that they have the new surgical procedure! Rachel's proctocolectomy will, hopefully, result in a continent (or pouch, or reservoir, or Kock) ileostomy; she will not have to wear an appliance; she will have the latest, the newest, the (Oh, God, please) barely-out-of-the-experimental stage procedure. "Don't think of it as losing your colon," Mark said to her a couple of days ago. "Think of it as gaining a pouch!"

The Germans have a much better word for what we call black humor: they call it *Galgenhumor*—gallows humor. So apt; it has been working overtime for us to keep us sane. Again we have reached the moment of seeing a child wheeled off to surgery, only she is not a child. She is twenty and adult and at the end of the road of almost twelve years of suffering and fighting a disease, and now she has won through to the decision that a sick colon can be traded for an altered status, for health. We kissed her, careful not to knock into the I.V. bottles. She said that we weren't to make it so damn tough on ourselves, go eat breakfast, do something, don't just sit there. A wobbly grin. "I'll be busy for a while."

What is probably the part of the poem I feel most strongly is the line about closing the heavy iron gate upon the colored images.

How easily I could have used all the colors in lurid symbolism. That's the way most of the poems of that period ran—four hundred of them written in one year of agony, a spilling, sputtering mess. However, they came before the acquired discipline of learning to write properly, and there are a few that survive. Now, after two published novels and some twenty stories in magazines good and bad, I am about to embark upon telling Rachel's story. At her urging. "Don't let it go to waste," she said, and of course I know what she meant—the lesson of living with a serious illness, the tale of not being stopped, the whole history of having come to this moment without feeling that we are defeated.

It is Rachel's victory primarily, but ours also. Sam's and Mark's and mine, and our other son, Daniel's, whose perspective was different. He has been free of the disease, and since he is much older, he was already out of the house when it all happened. We have never discussed what guilt he might have felt at being well and at being angry: Mark and I never did make it to any of his commencements together; we always had a sick child at home. But last time, when Dan and his wife, Ruth, and Davey and Beth, their children, came down from Boston to be with Rachel, it did not matter. All the feelings were somehow right: support and love and pain. Even the fury.

How did we get here? The long road. How did it start?

❧   ❧   ❧

During the summer of 1962 we were at the house in Hampton Bays on Long Island, as we had been since Sam's first year. A huge old wooden monstrosity standing in sixty-six acres of wilderness. Untamed grass, scrub pine, moss, blueberries, and poison ivy. The property abutted Shinnecock Bay, and there was blowing sand and seaweed and every kind of waving reed. Paradise to the children and Mark, a mixed blessing for me.

Yes, of course, it was beautiful; we used to see deer in the woods and hear the summer hum of bees and pick an orange weed—the name of which I never learned—that grew all over the wild meadow. It appeared right after the clumps of daisies had faded, and we filled every vase and jelly glass with it, and the children tanned and turned bronze. They looked like small Greek statues in their sun-bleached curls and perfect bodies. Mark taught them to dive through the breakers at the beach. A lovely sight, only it filled me with panic. The damn waves were huge and dangerous,

11

and Mark turns slightly manic in the ocean; I would stand there and shout, Be careful! Oh, puny understatement: are you crazy, Mark? They are so little. Though, really, it was comical, because normally Mark is the cautious one. When the children came out of the water, he insisted that they change into dry things. Not to catch colds.

Then there was my battle with the house, which was impossible to keep clean what with whispering sand in all the chinks and crunchy floors and the garbage pickup an uncertainty at best and the milk mostly sour at the stoop. The cesspool was finally located next to the front steps when the toilet paper came pushing up on the lawn next to them like the poppies in Flanders fields. Those were all the usual summer jokes, plus our private one: the blue Buick which was perhaps ten years old then. I can't understand anymore why it was *my* job to drive the hundred miles from New Jersey when it was Mark who couldn't part from the dear wreck because it had been his father's last car. Anyhow, when the tires weren't flat or the battery dead, we used to drive to the beach and go marketing in it. Mark also taught Sam to steer it, bumpety bump, across the sixty-six acres. "Nothing can happen to him here!" was his answer to my protest that nine was too young to drive.

Then there was the matter of help. The floor waxer did us on Thursday after the church. Except that he hardly ever showed up. And there was also the annual mother's helper. The previous summer she had been Swedish. She was not even all that pretty, with her long, thin, coltish legs, but a comet's tail of boys followed her as she walked along the beach with the kids—they were tossed high in the air by a lot of brawny arms that year, and they were not quite certain that they liked it. Surely I did not. Nor did the girl do much mother's helping. This year then, 1962, I had a Greek girl; we did not communicate so well, but she was homely.

Anyhow, it was a typical, wonderful summer. Dan, who was eighteen and about to go off to college, wrote from Israel that, believe it or not, he was debeaking chickens on the kibbutz and enjoying it. Sam—nine, and almost out of the cowboy stage—was into baseball and spent most of his time with the Berk boys, whose father, being a psychiatrist, had all of August free. He practiced togetherness with his kids via baseball rather than religion; Sam thought that was great. Rachel was six; roly-poly, a water rat, assertive. Except in thunderstorms. Then we took the kids into our beds and opened the blinds and showed them how beautiful the lightning was, how it lit up the night. Sam would say contemptuously, So what, and that he hadn't been afraid, but Rachel cuddled unashamedly. Anyhow, she was right: that wooden house would have flamed right to heaven if one of those gorgeous zigzags had come too close.

Still, after all the complaining was done, I knew that what I loved best was the sound of music that came into our beds at night. It came, softened by distance and water, from across the bay where the multi-rentals had raucous beer parties. But we were peaceful and safe and had special summer love.

And then Sam got violently ill with diarrhea and fever and terrible cramps. Of course it was Monday, after I had taken Mark to the train for his week at the office. "It must have been the appetizer last night," I said to him on the phone. We had been out for a fancy dinner on Sunday, and the appetizer had had a French name and uncertain paternity. Sam, who was a hamburger and French fries man, had hated it.

By Monday night, with his temperature climbing past 103 degrees, and with tough Sam suddenly looking all bones and angles, with sweat lying in the new hollows under his eyes, I got scared and insisted that the pediatrician come over. He said it was a virus and repeated that on the following day, but when the diarrhea turned bloody, he took tests while I kept rubbing Sam down with alcohol because the aspirin wouldn't control the fever.

At last the diagnosis: typhoid fever. Utterly bewildering, something archaic, like bubonic plague; how worried was I to be? I asked Ralph Berk, who told me that it was not what it used to be, that we had drugs now; Chloromycetin, he thought they'd use. "Lucky," he said; "I was afraid it was ulcerative colitis."

This last remark was not very meaningful to me, as I had never heard of ulcerative colitis, but it did sound reassuring: at least, typhoid fever was not the worst! In the meantime, we would all have to be inoculated to prevent an epidemic. It was amazing how many people had been in contact with Sam and were required to get two shots. The one who complained the most was the floor waxer, who had made one of his unusual appearances the previous Thursday.

Next came the Health Department. They questioned all of us and then informed me that our young helper might possibly be the typhoid carrier; that she had been exposed as a child and might or might not have had the fever. "I can't quite make it out," the Health Department man said. I wondered how he had gotten as much information as he had after I had ascertained that he spoke no Greek.

"Isn't there a test to determine whether or not someone is a carrier?" I inquired, and found that there was, only the girl refused to have it. Nor was there a way to press her into changing her mind. Or, for that matter, a way to fire her. With what seemed a kind of obtuse determination and with patient persistence, she made it clear that she had no other place to go, reminding me that I had hired her for the whole summer, and letting me know that if her fiancé were to find out about the possibility of her being a typhoid carrier, I would cause him to abandon her. ". . . he wants plenty children," she said. I ended up with a load of guilt to lug along with my resentment against her. One thing, however, was clear: I could not let her get close to beds, dishes, food, or Rachel. She spent the rest of the summer washing floors with Lysol and carrying water, because the Health Department had also condemned our well and our cesspool as possible sources of the infection.

Our landlord, who had become a friend over the many years of our tenantship, offered to split the cost of a cesspool and a brand-new well. But while the digging proceeded at an incredibly slow rate—"We can't dig in the rain, Missus"—there was nothing we could do but carry the water from an outdoor pump located halfway across the property. After taking our showers at friends' houses and then under a hose attached to the pump and finally, one awful Sunday when Sam kept sweating through pajamas at a mad rate, in a downpour of rain, Mark and I at last rented a room at a nearby motel for moments of peace and the use of a bathtub.

The sense of nightmare was growing. Our active, healthy Sam, also known as Tex, the fastest gun in the East, while always, each morning again, insisting that he was okay today, was practically shrinking away before our eyes. Three times a day we went through the ordeal of taking his temperature, which would not go down, and feeding him Chloromycetin as if it were candy, and somehow, each night, going to sleep thinking that by tomorrow the antibiotic would have taken hold, but all through the small hours hearing the racing footsteps to the bathroom, and knowing in the morning, just by looking at him, that he was not better.

Inevitably, I began to wonder whether it wasn't foolhardy not to hospitalize him. But it was impossible to decide. I accused myself of selfishness; I agonized that I was trying to escape this sense of panic; I was unprepared. Until then I had always been able to tolerate whatever anxiety accompanied the kids' sicknesses. They had had their usual share; all three had run high fevers with frequent sore throats. But it had never seemed reason for alarm. "Little kids run big temperatures," I would say to soothe Mark, who tended to be more apprehensive than I. Now, however, I was scared out of my wits. And it was Mark who tried to calm me down; reversed roles. Because this was out of my ken—this vicious pain that doubled Sam up, that made the perspiration pour off him, that forced the moans between his clenched teeth. And all that blood. He took care to come out of the bathroom humming and nonchalant—though the pajama jacket stuck to his ribs; though I saw the concentration it took to walk normally.

And most of all: the doctor! There was no doubt that he was bewildered, that this diarrhea, this typhoid fever, did not respond as had been expected. While he had at first insisted that a hospitalization would mean that Sam would have to be isolated in an infectious-disease unit, and that the danger of his catching something horrible there was greater than the risk involved in keeping him at home, he seemed not to be so sure of that anymore. He was consulting with colleagues in New York.

It's hard to remember now how Rachel fared during that time. Though, of course, some events stand out. Her resistance to the typhoid inoculation has become family lore: the doctor and I chasing the screaming child around the dining-room table! And I recall—just a few frames out of a strip of film—the sight of her sitting on the front steps one drizzly day, sitting on her hands, making spit bubbles. "You okay?" I inquired, passing her, lugging yet another pail of water. "When's Sam coming down to play?" she whined. What I did then is obscured by the memory of a red tide of anger that swept me. Couldn't Rachel see what was going on? What was the matter with her? Smart kid of six, did she have to pull this baby act on me now? Probably I yelled at her.

Another thing I remember is that Rachel enjoyed a triumphal ride back to town in the front of the ambulance. The driver let her sound the siren.

Not so Sam. It was after his fever had finally gone down, after these almost four weeks of constantly veering between a hundred two and three. But he was still terribly sick, bleeding profusely, in much pain and exceedingly weak. The doctor definitely wanted him off the Chloromycetin; in fact, he wanted out of this bizarre case. So it was agreed that Presbyterian Medical Center would accept Sam into Babies Hospital. The pediatrician who would take over, a Dr. Sanford Burns, had an excellent reputation, we were told. Several telephone consultations, during which we talked a lot and he maintained grave silence but for hm's and ahh's, had somehow convinced us that he was a man of wisdom, experience, and prestige; he would have the answers. And we needed answers, because now Sam's typhoid fever tests were coming back negative. And God, we needed to be reassured!

So I rode with Sam in the back of the ambulance. My attempts to present our ride as an adventure—"Look at us, sirens screaming in the night, red lights flashing!"—fell flat. Sam asked me to pull the shades down; he did not want anyone to see him, to feel sorry for him, to think perhaps he wasn't tough. He wished that the dumb Rachel would stop the racket, stop calling attention to us.

"Sam, don't be a dolt," I argued. "People get sick; it's no disgrace."

He shrugged. Clearly, I did not understand. Cowboys, and for that matter, baseball players, did not have diseases, certainly not embarrassing ones like diarrhea. It had been different last year when he had suffered from a six-week bout of osteomyelitis. That illness, while also somewhat shameful because it necessitated crutches, had at least been something he had in common with a number of sports heroes.

No, Sam did not enjoy the ambulance ride.

❦ ❦ ❦

MARCH 4, 1977

Noon

Sam is reading a tome that says CONTRACTS on the spine. He underlines in yellow; he seems absorbed. Mark is also working. An inventory-control chart is spread across his knees; he is shaking his head at the figures he examines. And I have lain down on Rachel's bed and turned on the heating pad. It feels good; I realize suddenly how much my back hurts from the tension in which I have been holding myself. I try to relax my muscles, then quickly sit up as a nurse walks in, feeling embarrassed. Maybe I shouldn't be on the bed—contamination from my street clothes? The nurse stashes some surgical supplies on one of the shelves. I make a little joke, say that I'm the new patient, and she smiles, and Mark and Sam look up and smile as well. Then it is quiet again.

Lying here, I see the room from Rachel's perspective, as she saw it yesterday, will see it tomorrow when she comes back; the doctor has explained that she will stay in the recovery room overnight. It is a large room, bright, with a view of Central Park. The feeling of familiarity I have as I look around is underscored by the fact that it's the identical room I had, two or three floors below, when Rachel was born. Yes, right here in Klingenstein Pavilion I had my first sight of her and experienced instant love for this completely unexpected girl child; Mark and I had taken another boy for granted, had neither wanted a girl nor picked a name for her. And then the nurse had walked in with this tiny Buddha-faced person and some completely new emotion had burst open in me . . . fantastic, a Rachel.

I think of it now as I look at the forest of hanging plants on the I.V. poles we have abducted from a supply closet and at the posters we've put up. There is one I found of a kitten on a chinning bar. It says, "Hang in there, Baby." Something in the small grave cat face is very moving, and a wave of fear courses through me: oh, God, perhaps too well chosen a poster; who needs inspirational messages from a Japanese chain named Azuma? I turn away from it.

The windowsills are lined with books; Rachel is expecting to be able to work on her research paper in a few days. I have to grin remembering one of the doctors walking in and examining the titles and getting very uncomfortable until Rachel explained that her preoccupation with death and dying is academic. After he left, we went hysterical. Oh, did you see his face? Oh, a patient checking in for surgery with twenty books on dying. Too much!

"What are you laughing about?" Mark asks. But it's too much trouble to explain and suddenly doesn't seem funny anymore, and I say, Nothing, and all three of us look at our watches. If they started punctually at eight . . . no, we can't possibly hear anything until four o'clock. "Let's go for some coffee," Mark suggests, and though I'd rather stay right here, right here on Rachel's bed, I know that is stupid and helps no one. Nor will it hurry time.

In the elevator I ask them, "Do you remember Dr. Burns?"

Sam answers, "Ah, Mom!" He says it in the same annoyed tone he used to employ if I stepped on forbidden territory when he was a kid. Ah, Mom! Don't be sentimental, don't be sappy, don't mix up my baseball cards. Today: don't regurgitate the past. Maybe he is right. In fact, he is certainly right for himself. That's his way of coping, at least outwardly: let's not talk about it.

But for me the need to look back, to examine, to understand is imperative. If I can get it orderly in my mind, in sequence, how it was . . .

❧ ❧ ❧

That first hospitalization at Presbyterian. Sam refusing the wheelchair, walking the long corridor, his skinny shoulder blades. And Dr. Burns. Dr. Burns informed us that he did not think that Sam had typhoid fever. "Does not have it now, or never had it?" A shrug. It was difficult to deal with Dr. Burns; he did not talk a lot; his eyes were cold, though Sam said that he was friendly to him when we were not around. Mark and I figured that he had nothing to say to us; they were making tests. At least they didn't require us to put on sterile gowns anymore. After the first few days, we could just walk into Sam's room, and he was allowed to have company. Except that he didn't want any. Emphatically, he did not want his friends to know he was sick. Grandma? Okay, if she must, but Tommy, no. "I'll see him when I get home." Tomorrow. It was always tomorrow, or certainly in a few days.

And then the doctor actually talked about discharging him. Very officially, in his office from behind his desk, a veritable stream of words: the stool cultures had shown neither amebic nor bacillary dysentery, and all the other tests had also been negative, but of course, these gastroenteritis things were often nonspecific, and the picture was further obscured by the use of the Chloromycetin. With a little note of accusation and a shake of the head: "Heavy guns, Chloromycetin!"

I listened and nodded; I looked over at Mark, who was also nodding as if hypnotized. But, I thought, is Sam better? Is he all right? Why does he still bleed? However, there was no pause in Dr. Burns's presentation during which I might have asked these questions. And it was as if we were brainwashed into a sort of helplessness, that we were compelled to simply concentrate on what the man said about a bland diet, a milder antibiotic, and that it might take a while longer until the symptoms disappeared. "These things do," Dr. Burns said. These things? Then, magnanimously, "And you can take young Samson home tomorrow."

I actually said, "Oh, thank you, Doctor."

Outside, Mark and I did not look at each other.

So we took Sam home. It worked out just right, because Mark had to make an urgent business trip to Europe and had been putting it off as long as Sam was in the hospital. We had a proper celebration before he left: Sam was home; after all, we said; they would not have discharged him if he were not on the way to recovery. But the first night after Mark had left, at all hours, I heard Sam. And lay open-eyed in the dark, realizing that I had forgotten during the time he had been "safe" in the hospital what heavy apprehension those racing footsteps in the night evoked. And lay pondering the question whether to get up and offer help or to stay in bed and pretend not to hear and in the morning nod and smile when Sam would say that he was much better. In the end I stayed in bed. Opting for his dignity over comfort? I was not sure. Nor am I now, looking back. How much did I take my cues from the children; how much did I impose my needs on them? In any case, in the morning I took Rachel to school and then was back with Sam. It was a gray day; his skin was gray too; his eyes were huge. We played "Sorry."

All through the weeks of illness I had been in touch with Dr. Curt Freeman, our New Jersey pediatrician, on the telephone. Since he was also connected with Presbyterian, I had been reassured by his endorsement of Dr. Burns. And that evening, when Sam's temperature suddenly shot up, we had a long conversation. "Do you know whether they tested him for ulcerative colitis?" he asked at one point. I said no, I did not, that I'd never heard it mentioned. Yet it had a familiar ring. Oh, yes: Ralph Berk's remark that day in the summer. Quickly, I turned my mind away from that recollection and said, "Please, Curt, will you see Sam in the morning?" He promised that he would. He would also speak to Dr. Burns. I felt better having him officially on the case. And before going to bed, I filled out a coupon I had recently clipped: I ordered the *New Illustrated Medical Encyclopaedia For Home Use*. It was time for me to be better informed.

Dr. Freeman saw Sam the next day and the day after. Sam was again in terrible pain, bleeding, unable to eat. Curt sat by his bedside after feeling his belly, listening through his stethoscope, holding Sam's wrist, patting his arm. Outside, he said to me that he wanted him back in the hospital, that he had suggested some tests to Dr. Burns that had not been made the last time.

"But can't we have them done on an outpatient basis? Can't you do them?"

"I could, but I'd rather he be at the hospital."

I didn't argue. Dr. Curt Freeman was not an alarmist.

"I'll tell him," he said, and walked back into Sam's room.

Sam made only one demand: no ambulance this time. I was acutely aware, on the way to the hospital, that we had dead silence in the car as we drove across the George Washington Bridge. But somehow I could not subject Sam to assurances and inanities. When we were almost there, he asked me whether I would tell Mark that he was back in the hospital. I stalled by replying that Daddy might not call that night. But when Sam insisted, I asked him whether he wanted me to tell. "No," Sam said firmly. "No, don't. There's nothing he can do from Italy; he'll just worry."

"Well, he'll be back Friday." We were stopped for a light. I looked at Sam, at his drawn expression, and suddenly knew that I was doing this all wrong. "No, wait a minute," I said hastily. "I don't think that Dad would like to be treated as if he were a fragile old lady."

"But why worry him? There's nothing he can *do!*" His tone was sharp now.

"Just the same," I insisted.

Sam shrugged. Then he looked out his window. He managed it by rotating his body in such a manner that his back was turned to me. An angry back; oh, Sam.

This time he was put into a children's ward. An enormous, long room; Sam's bed was at the end, next to a window. Across from him was Philip, whose mother said that he had C.F. It took a long time until he gathered enough breath to say hello to Sam.

Later, after leaving punctually at the end of visiting hours, I was oppressed that I had been persuaded to go along with having Sam on the ward. The reasons presented to me were that it was psychologically better for a child to be with his peers, that it would lessen dependence on parents (an obvious virtue!), and that it was more cheerful. All of which had made sense to me in theory, but now I wondered. How cheerful was it to listen to Philip? Certainly *I* had tried my best all afternoon not to hear his agonizing struggle to bring up phlegm. What was C.F., anyhow? Cheerful! Unless, by comparison? No.

And Sam had been angry at me. Was it because I had taken him back to the hospital or because of the ward? Or because he would have to go through a series of x-rays and tests and procedures the next day? An intern had explained the program to us, but I was not clear on all he had said. I had sat and tried to look alert, but inside I had felt only panic at the unfamiliar terms, at going through this without Mark, at having set machinery in motion that suddenly seemed evil. Like the sorcerer's apprentice, I thought. As to Sam, apparently he had attended better. In any case, he had asked many questions which the young doctor had answered carefully; then they had discussed the Yankees. When the nurse announced the end of visiting hours, Sam had said, "But Daddy always stays till nine."

"They won't let me, here." I had apologized.

"Yeah, I know," he had said. But he had been angry at me.

Which was nothing compared with the way he felt when I got there the next day. A furious boy, expressions on his face I did not know. Not easygoing, not funny, not Sam. Furious. Sitting in a detested wheelchair, he had apparently been kept waiting for two hours in the x-ray department. And where had I been? He hadn't even had a book to read. Boy, if he had known that it would take that long, he could have taken his stamps along; he could have pasted in all the new African ones. But he had just sat there, waiting and waiting in that dumb chair. Why did they take him down to x-ray if they weren't ready for him? And some dumb nurse had given him a comic. "Superman!" Sam's voice spat with contempt.

I tried to explain that visiting hours didn't start till two; he didn't listen.

"And that dumb lab technician!" She had stuck him several times before getting blood, which, of course, he didn't care about —it didn't even hurt—but afterward Dr. Greer (yesterday's intern, Sam's friend now) had said that she'd done all the wrong tests; they'd have to get blood for the right ones tomorrow. "And when Dr. Santiago examined me, he had three student nurses watching!" Sam's face was distorted, perspiration on his upper lip, his voice, though low, strident.

I wanted to apologize. Oh, Sam, I'm sorry. Yes, why hadn't I been there to prevent all those mishaps, to keep him company, to save him? Except that I knew that my presence would not have made the least difference. This was not my milieu; here I was not Mommy who blows away hurts; in fact, half the time I didn't even understand what Sam was talking about. What blood tests? And who was Dr. Santiago? I ventured the latter question. Sam said impatiently that he was the surgeon Dr. Greer had told us about yesterday—didn't I remember?

At last his fury had run its course and Sam grinned. "Sorry."

Relieved, I launched into the story of my morning. First thing, I had received a call from Rachel's teacher asking me to come over during lunch recess, and when I had gotten there—

Sam interrupted. "Did you tell her about me?" Miss Williams had been Sam's first-grade teacher as well.

"She knew from Rachel. But of course she wanted to hear what it was. I told her that we're waiting for a diagnosis, but that it is not typhoid."

"Okay. But don't tell everyone. And Dr. Burns wants to see you at four."

I felt a wave of heat in my stomach, but said calmly, "Well, thanks for telling me." And when Sam looked stubborn, I continued, "Do you want to hear about Rachel?"

"Sure."

"Well, Miss Williams started in very gently—about how she knows what nice, smart children I have . . ."

"But?"

"But Rachel refuses to read. She looks at her book, and then she beams at Miss Williams and says that she doesn't know what it says."

Sam guffawed.

I began to embroider the story, giving Miss Williams some additional lines of praise for Sam and myself several witticisms. However, I left out the part where we had decided that this lack of performance was Rachel's bid for attention. But Sam was way ahead of me. He said that it was obvious that Rachel could read this junk in the baby reader with her eyes closed, that he had taught it to her himself when he had learned it, and that she was just angry because I spent all my time with him. He made this declaration in a mixture of annoyance and pride, apparently taking some pleasure in her obstinacy, but also impatient with me for falling into Rachel's trap.

"Well, Miss Williams and I decided that some homework will fix her. If she is suddenly required to do extra work, she might find it more convenient to read." I looked at my watch: another hour until I'd see Dr. Burns. "Want me to get you some ice cream?"

"No. They haven't told me yet what I can eat. Because of the x-rays."

"What? Again? I thought they did them today."

"Maybe they'll need more."

We sat staring at each other. I wanted terribly to ask him whether he knew anything I did not, but there was a veiled look, something forbidding. At the same time his expression, his very posture—a skinny pile of boy in the middle of the bed—cried out for comfort. But when I reached to hug him, he pushed my arm away and looked over my shoulder at Philip, who was sleeping. Such touch me, touch me not; I felt my throat close up, began to cough. Then I had to lean close to hear what Sam said next. "You'll tell me everything he says!" Without a question mark.

"I promise."

After which he let me take his hand.

By the time Dr. Burns told me that Sam had ulcerative colitis, I had wiped Ralph's remark of the summer out of my mind and remembered only that this was what Dr. Freeman had suggested. Dr. Burns switched on a panel of lights and showed me a number of x-rays—swollen, milky sausages. Since I had no basis for comparing these portraits of Sam's intestines with a set of healthy ones, Dr. Burns's pointing ruler meant very little to me. What I understood, however, was that Dr. Santiago's clinical findings had confirmed the diagnosis. I further learned that we were not dealing with a gastroenteritis, as Dr. Burns had first suspected, and that ulcerative colitis was not to be confused with spastic colitis, which is often attributed to nerves. Dr. Burns cleared his throat, said, "I presume that you have heard of children who react to every emotional upheaval with bouts of diarrhea!" His voice was contemptuous.

But no, unfortunately, we were dealing with an entirely different illness: with an organic form of colitis which was grave indeed. A serious inflammatory disease of the large bowel—he pointed at the x-rays again. I looked at them dutifully, uncomprehendingly. Dr. Burns's delivery, I noted, was a monotone. Words like bloody diarrhea, general weakness, joint involvement, pain, retardation of growth and arrest of sexual development . . . just words; they fell evenly, unemphatically, undifferentiated. And he was looking straight at me, but I had no sense of being seen.

"What is the treatment?" I asked.

He sat back in his chair. I thought he looked relieved—which

23

alerted me. Why? Because I had not made a fuss? Was a fuss in order? What was I missing? I repeated, my voice sharper, "I mean, what kind of treatment is indicated? How long will it take?"

There was no telling. Also, relapses were to be expected; but, fortunately, very good results were being attained with steroids. He added quickly, "Small doses, conservative doses."

Sensing danger here, I dug in. "Steroids?" I asked. "Like cortisone? Isn't that a very dangerous drug?" I thought indignantly that he had shaken his head at the use of Chloromycetin.

Dr. Burns was becoming impatient with me. "Of course, of course these are potent drugs, and there are undesirable side effects, but I did explain to you that we would put young Samson on a very conservative dose. I think you will find that steroids have great therapeutic value."

"What kind of substance are they?" I asked, in spite of the fact that Burns had risen. There was a bee swarm of story fragments in my mind, awful things I had heard . . .

He was walking to the door, and I too had risen. Now his voice was back to the monotone. Actually, he explained, the body produces cortisone from the adrenal glands; we would simply bolster the natural process with some additional synthetic product. And I would see, yes, probably quite a dramatic improvement.

Then I was in the corridor. Neat, I thought; oh, neat! It seemed to me, though, that I had ducked away from a hand raised to pat my shoulder reassuringly. I hoped so. I headed straight for the telephone booth and called Dr. Freeman, but the nurse would not let me through. "Mrs. Bergman, this office is a madhouse today," she said jovially, certain of my understanding. "He'll get back to you later." I said sure, okay. And stood there, the background sounds I had just heard still in my ears—a baby crying, someone's laughter, a child's shout. A great longing swept me: to be there, to be in the familiar pediatrician's office, to hold Sam in my lap, Sam at six months for a checkup, Sam at two . . . is it measles? Sam having something normal, known.

Back on the ward, Sam was playing checkers with the boy from two beds down. He said, "This is Bob. He has arthritis." And then, looking up once more, "Hey, Dr. Greer says I don't have to have more tests! They know what it is. It's called ulcerative colitis. It's an inflammation in the large bowel." He watched my face.

"I know." Easy, easy; if I can't reach Curt Freeman tonight, whom can I call? Who will explain? Our cousin Gustav, Gustl? He was a dermatologist, but he would know. And be upset, and not want to worry me . . . no. I asked, "Do you boys want some ice cream?"

"Oh, boy, can I have chocolate?" Bob shouted.

"Vanilla." And Sam added, "I'm going to get the same medicine Bob has to take. It's called Prednisone."

"Oh? I thought Dr. Burns said steroids. Or maybe cortisone."

The boy Bob laughed uproariously. I saw that his back buckled under the right shoulder. He grabbed Sam's hand. "Oh, she's funny, funny!" And to me, "Prednisone is the trade name. It *is* cortisone, which is a steroid, see?"

I nodded.

But Sam turned on Bob, his voice angry, "You think you're so smart. Who wants to know all that junk?"

"I know all about drugs," the boy boasted, and added, "I've been sick for nine years."

"That's how old I am," Sam blurted.

"I'm twelve." He looked no bigger than Sam.

"Okay," I said hastily. "One chocolate and one vanilla coming up." My footsteps clicked on the vinyl floor.

Curt Freeman called me at ten o'clock. "Too late for you?"

"God, no." Basically he didn't add much to Dr. Burns's explanation, but I could ask questions. I listened while he also said that ulcerative colitis was a serious inflammatory disease of the colon, which was another name for the large bowel, and that Dr. Santiago had seen typical signs of the disease during the proctoscopy: namely, bleeding produced by slight rubbing of the walls of the sigmoid and even up higher—"

"What's the sigmoid?" I interrupted to ask.

"The lower portion of the large bowel."

"Colon!"

"Yes."

"Go on," I urged.

"There isn't much else. It will all depend on how serious Sam's case is. Many children suffer only minor periodic episodes."

"But what is the cure?"

"We don't have a cure. Nor do we know the cause. Fairly good results have been attained with conservative doses of adrenal steroids and some of the salicylazosulfapyridine-type drugs." He hesitated, then added, "And there's quite a dispute on the question of diet. Some of the newer authorities do not go along with the importance of a bland diet without roughage which was the old standby."

I listened with growing unease. Curt was being terribly careful. Once he interrupted to ask when Mark would be back. Finally I willed myself to ask, "But what if Sam has a bad case? And what about all that business with retardation?" Suddenly I was unbearably anxious. I cried out, "I don't understand! What connection can there be between a disease of the colon and not growing and developing?"

"Look, Jean, listen!" Yes, Curt was disturbed. He said I was upsetting myself needlessly. He said, "There's no sense scaring yourself with every dire possibility. Let's take it a step at a time. Let's first see how Sam reacts to the Prednisone."

"Okay." I was ready to agree. Yes, he was right. Of course he was right. I listened as he spoke reassuringly about the excellence of Babies Hospital and the competence of Dr. Burns.

"Except that it was you who had to tell him what to look for before he could make a diagnosis," I replied bitterly.

"That's silly," Curt demurred modestly, and he made a little joke about the last doctor always being the smartest.

At last I let him hang up. Not feeling better, or smarter.

MARCH 4, 1977

3 P.M.

It is no longer possible to stay busy. Sam is looking out the window; how it rains! Mark is pacing. I can't take my eyes off the charcoal drawing Rachel did about a year ago. It is of a baby being born; square rubber fingers cradle its head. Its eyes are still closed, but there is a look of concentration, maybe of determination, around the mouth—it is almost awake, almost born, trembling between here and there. Rachel came across the drawing just recently and showed it to me. I asked whether I could have it, and she gave it to me. However, after I had it framed, when Rachel was already in the hospital, I offered to lend it back to her for the duration.

Neither of us expressed why it seemed so appropriate to put a nail into the wall of this room and hang it up, but now it is perfectly clear to me why it touched us, why we named it "Rebirth" when "Birth" would be a more accurate title. And I suddenly understand the degree of awareness with which Rachel has gone into this surgery. The fact that she has more than ordinary knowledge of the process is due not only to this affinity she has for things medical, nor just because she asked every possible question and insisted on the answers; it is because she has really faced the emotional ramifications as well. As I think that, my courage deserts me, and I shy away from the thought, I want to deny it . . . no, she cannot, I think, not consciously, she cannot consciously have identified with this baby's push to emerge. And then argue: Why not? How else could she have made the decision?

Then the door opens and there is Dr. David Gaon. It is like an explosion of joy. How does he manage to say all the longed-for things at once, immediately, simultaneously—that she is fine, that everything went according to the book, that he found no malignancy, that he was able to establish the internal pouch, that she has the continent ileostomy? And yes, the surgery was very necessary. Standing there in his operating greens down to the booties, with his hair tousled, exuding warmth, the most beautiful man in the world. Mark and Sam are shaking his hand; we are all laughing, laughing.

"It had to go splendidly," Dr. Gaon says. "The last thing she told me before going under was that she listened to the whole Megillah last night." Yes, it is Purim today, the celebration of the rescue of the Jews from Haman's plot to destroy them. The Megillah, traditionally written on a scroll, is read each year in commemoration. It is considered a good deed to read it and to listen to it; Rachel wasn't going to miss that. "And she washed her hair too," I say, and we laugh some more.

After Dr. Gaon leaves, we cry. We hug each other and cry. And I try not to think of what is immediately ahead, of pain, of the climb back which is yet to be accomplished by Rachel. I try to join in the euphoria Sam and Mark seem to be feeling. They keep saying that it is over. Thank God, they say, it is over. And we keep holding each other.

❧ ❧ ❧

The first I knew of an ileostomy was when I read about it in the *New Medical Encyclopaedia for Home Use.* It had arrived while I had gone to the hospital to pick up Sam. It was three weeks later and Sam was Sam again, restored, healed; he was putting back the lost weight.

"It's just as you said: a dramatic improvement!" I had said in our final conversation with Dr. Burns, who had suddenly been less unpleasant. I had thanked him for all he had done for Sam, and said that it was amazing how quickly Sam had begun to get better after starting the Prednisone. "He's himself again," I had said to Dr. Burns. "In fact, he's even making jokes about the speed with which he used to make it to the bathroom." Dr. Burns nodded, though I could see that he was astonished at the way I was gushing after the chilliness that had marked our relationship. Yes, he agreed, the boy was very much improved, but we were to be prepared for a possible relapse. "Of course," I replied politely, and attributed this petty carping on the unthinkable to the man's terrible personality; really! Thank goodness, this would be the last of him. The ride home had been pure triumph, and the front door had been adorned with a WELCOME HOME sign. Upstairs, on Sam's bed, was a new baseball glove. We had roast beef for dinner and Sam ate two helpings.

So what made me go down to the study after the children and even Mark were asleep? What made me unwrap the bulky package and search the four volumes of the Medical Encyclopaedia for information on ulcerative colitis? And do it with my heart pounding palpably in my throat, with a feeling of sickness in my belly; do it furtively like a child who has found the sex manual under her mother's nightgowns? It is hard to say in retrospect, but I do remember that I slammed the book shut indignantly when I read the passage about surgery. And then climbed on a chair and pushed the box with the green books way back on the top shelf of the bookcase. It serves me right, I fumed: reading trashy layman's books on medicine. "For Home Use" indeed! Written for the ignorant, for idiots like me. The whole thing was preposterous. It said that chances for recovery from ulcerative colitis were excellent provided surgery is performed at an appropriate time. Utter humbug. Neither Curt Freeman nor Dr. Burns had mentioned anything about surgery. And the book further stated that people with permanent ileostomies learn to manage effectively and perform all the functions of the normal. The normal! They must be kidding.

On the way to bed I made a firm resolution to forget the whole nonsense; specifically to forget the drawings the book had provided. Sam was well now. All I had to do to know that was look at him. I stood by his bed and pulled up his covers; he was tall, sturdy, sleeping fiercely, happily back in his own bed. The new glove was on his night table; he and Rachel had celebrated his return with a terrific fight already.

We did not get much of a respite. Two months later, in November, Sam came home at noon one day.

"Hooky or half day?" I inquired.

He mumbled about not feeling well and sped upstairs. I tried to stay at my typewriter, but couldn't make it. Sam lay in bed facing the wall. I sat down next to him, put a hand on his shoulder. "Tell me?" I asked.

He turned around; he had not been crying. "What's to tell?" Then, with satisfaction, "No one noticed. I told the office I had a sore throat."

"But it's your belly?"

"Yes."

"When did it start?"

"A couple of days ago. But not bad; there was no blood."

"But now there is."

"Just a little." Then, pushing me roughly aside, he was out of bed, sprinting to the bathroom, slamming the door.

And I sat, hands in lap, listening. I don't believe that I was thinking, or suffering. Just resting before having to get involved.

Dr. Freeman sent us to a specialist in New Haven because none of us wanted more of Dr. Burns. Dr. Irving Samuelson was a nice, comfortable man who told Sam immediately not to worry, he would not sigmoidoscope him, he didn't believe in it. So we all liked him immediately. Then we talked and he studied the x-rays and he examined Sam, whose shoulder blades were prominent again. "I'll tell you my philosophy on ulcerative colitis," he declared. We listened carefully.

Later, when Mark and I tried to recollect, it was difficult to decide what his philosophy was. Finally, I summed it up. "He said we were not to look into the toilet bowl!"

"Well, that's hardly all he said," Mark demurred.

"But that was the final message."

"In other words, there isn't much that can be done. There's no cure, no known cause, and he doesn't believe in the use of steroids."

"He said to use them only sparingly, for short periods. That he'd direct Curt Freeman . . ." I broke off, thought. Then added,

29

"The feeling I got was that he said Curt knows as little as anyone else, so we might as well use him!"

"He didn't say that!"

"No, but he left me with the impression."

"And what was that about surgery? What did he say about surgery?"

I repeated the doctor's words verbatim: "He said, 'These cases either come to surgery or not'!" I didn't elaborate.

We were sitting in the study, drinking tea. I looked up at the bookshelf. Then I shrugged. I had observed during the consultation that neither Mark nor I reacted to the remark the doctor made about surgery. And thought that at least *I* was cognizant of my refusal to deal with this. Oh, but I felt a great shock at the word "surgery," a shock and a surprise because, indeed, I had completely forgotten about what was said in the stupid book. Nor did Mark seem to want to explore the subject further now. He said bitterly, "Well, if he's the great expert on ulcerative colitis, they don't know much." He also said that he wouldn't leave it at that. He would find out. Next week in Europe, in Switzerland, in England, in Russia . . . someplace they must have some answers.

So Mark went on his odyssey, disguised as a business trip, and Sam followed the medical regimen prescribed by Dr. Freeman via Dr. Samuelson. I have forgotten what the exact dose of Prednisone was, but I recall that it was not enough to produce as spectacular a "cure" as it had the previous time. But Sam was able to go back to school, more or less well.

Only there was a crack in our sense of invincibility.

CHAPTER *2*

RACHEL, AGE 16:

When I was six years old my brother became very ill. For a while we thought that he would die. In retrospect, there appears to be no way that I could have failed to realize the seriousness of the situation; yet, conveniently, I did. Of course now I see that my behavior expressed a lot of anger; I was convinced that my parents loved my brother better and I accused them of this repeatedly until I succeeded in provoking the scene which gave me the attention I craved: out of exasperation and helplessness, my mother finally exploded. She asked me how I could be so selfish and insensitive, and didn't I realize that when she and my brother went off every day it was not for their pleasure; they were going to doctors. She asked whether it was possible that I did not understand how sick my brother was.

I will never forget the feeling of shock and disbelief I felt at that moment, not to mention the shame. Afterwards it seemed inappropriate for me to go about my own affairs without a constant feeling of guilt and sorrow, and I recognized all the things I had not previously allowed myself to comprehend. And yet, this did not change my behavior in the least. I still fussed over going to school and refused to learn to read. And as to my thoughts about God, I decided that He was far from benevolent if he allowed such a thing to happen to a child.

Well, my brother lived. But in my mind this period is closely associated with death; certainly, three years later when I found that I had the same disease, I felt great concern for my continuing existence.

MARCH 4, 1977

7 P.M.

Dr. Gaon has stopped by once more and told us that Rachel is doing well. He said we could take a quick peek at her in the recovery room after six o'clock.

We have traversed the underground corridors following the black signs to the Annenberg Pavilion; we have taken the escalator up into the impressive black marble lobby of this latest addition to the Mt. Sinai complex of buildings old and new, and we have searched for the elevator that will take us to the sixth floor. Twice we found cars in which the "6" was blacked out; at last we locate the one that will stop at the recovery room. I can't breathe, choked with anxiety; I want to be there, be with Rachel, and I want to hide, to send Mark instead. I want to cower with my hands covering my head. I am prepared for the sight of the tubes and catheters, the monitors, the I.V.s; I am prepared for the smell of blood; and I am totally unprepared.

A nice young man shows us the sterile gowns and booties we are to wear. "Two at a time, not more than ten minutes altogether," he directs. I follow the robed Mark into the giant room, feeling as if I walk a corridor with walls of white sound on both sides, curtains of beeps swelling into a roar. I know and don't know that there are other beds, other moans, and I am not sure whether the pounding is my blood.

Here is Rachel. She is awake, terribly awake and alert; she is in total agony. Mark bends close to her cracked lips. She asks whether she has the pouch, whether the surgery was necessary, whether the pathology report is back. Mark and I talk fast, telling her all the good things Dr. Gaon has said. I hold her hand; Mark strokes the hair out of her face. We repeat over and over, brightly, that everything went well, that Dr. Gaon says the pouch works beautifully. "You're fine, fine," we say.

Rachel speaks normally but as if distracted: "It hurts, it hurts dreadfully. I didn't think it would hurt like this. My back, ohh . . ." her voice going out of control; tears roll down her cheeks. Mark answers that she will get more painkillers, they won't let her suffer, they'll make her comfortable. "I just got morphine; it doesn't help," she protests, but Mark replies that it will, it will in a minute. Suddenly my ears are roaring, I break into a sweat, nausea wells up. I let go of Rachel's hand and turn and see a chair at the nurses' island in the middle of the room. Concentrating, I make it over there. Then the young man is pushing my head down.

In the car driving home I'm still fighting nausea, still feeling the rapid pulse, still bitterly ashamed.

"Stop worrying." Mark tries to calm me. "I told her that they only allow two people in, that it was Sam's turn. She didn't notice."

But of course that isn't the point. The point is the pain—why are they letting her have so much pain? Why is the pain so bad in her back? "Maybe we should call Dr. Gaon?" I ask.

Mark assures me that he heard the intern call him and ask permission to increase the morphine, that the intern told Gaon how alert she was. . . .

"Look," Sam interjects, "that's why they're keeping her in the recovery room overnight. So they can monitor the pain and make her comfortable. We just hit a bad minute. By now she's way under. . . ."

Mark agrees.

I realize that they're talking fast to keep their own panic down, and I don't protest their illogic, don't say: you know that's bull, you know they can't give her more, they need her alert so that she'll breathe deeply, will move around, will do all the things for which they need her cooperation. I don't say it, but it is all over my mind, my body, my soul. All the day's discipline has evaporated, the colored images are out from behind the heavy iron gate, all the careful calm is caught in the rotation of the crazy centrifuge that is my insides. Oh, God, please God, don't let her suffer like that.

❦   ❦   ❦

Rachel's recollections of Sam's illness do not really match mine; and while it may appear from her account that Mark and I understood the seriousness, the very life-or-death quality of his condition, the fact is that we faced it no better than she did.

We went on a cruise on the S.S. *France* that winter. Sam was what Dr. Freeman and Dr. Samuelson called "in remission." I think that, this being so, I was perhaps a little resentful because he didn't enjoy the trip. He hated the fancy meals, for which he had no appetite whatever, and he was annoyed with Rachel, who relished everything from ordering caviar to getting dressed up in party frocks for dinner and who took to all the luxury as if it were her natural habitat. Sam said contemptuously that she was disgusting. But mostly he hated the stops at the islands, with their swarm of children descending on him to beg for nickels.

Mark and I discussed it, and we did understand that the contrasts were too much for him, that it mortified him to be the rich kid from the fancy ship. But what I don't think we comprehended was that Sam identified with the young beggars. To us Sam was still the triumphant child—the beautiful, the smart, the tall boy; I believe now that the experience of the illness was changing his self-image. And in a way he was being more realistic than we were, because he was every bit as skinny, as scrawny, as drawn-looking as the native children and undoubtably, even in "remission," he was not feeling really well. I seem to remember only one time that Sam had fun on that trip; in any case his eyes were shining and he had a broad smile as he watched a shapely dancer with an enormous diamond in her belly button do gyrations on Curaçao, in the Netherlands Antilles.

Each child has its place in the family constellation; we always thought of Sam as being best situated.

Daniel is, of course, my firstborn, but he was also the one whose mother was nineteen when he arrived on the scene. I was still playing house then, and the baby was my treasured toy. I had to do a lot of growing up before I was able to see a child as an individual separate from myself. And then he went through my divorce with me. Although he was only three when Mark came into our lives, he experienced the usual upheavals of the child with several sets of parents.

As to Rachel, her being a girl had made her my sister as well as my child. We are very different in some ways, but I always feel admiration for her, though sometimes reluctantly, and even when we are in conflict I can at least understand her. But she was born into a difficult time in our lives and was still very small when Mark's father died and both Mark and I came unglued; life without Papa was very rough for a while.

Sam, however, had come at the perfect moment, at the very height of our readiness to have a child together and at a moment we deemed to be right for Dan to accept a sibling. So he was surrounded by a very good quality of love from the beginning, love from all of us—Dan and Mark and me and that grandfather whose lovingness was an extraordinary thing.

Sam was a dignified and self-contained child, setting limits, demanding respect; somehow one didn't talk baby nonsense to Sam. But he was also gay and loving and incredibly good-looking—dark eyes and blond curls—yet tough. Named Joshua Samson Bergman, it was he who chose to be called Sam (it went with the low-slung holsters), and even his grandmothers had to accept the change from Joshy to Sam. And he was bright, which helped during the next years when he began to miss a lot of school.

At first I was not really aware of the changes in his life. Sam's natural reticence made it seem normal that he didn't want his friends to know about the illness, that he didn't even want to discuss it with us. During remissions he joined his fellows in every kind of sport and fun; part of a trio known as "the terrible three," he spent a lot of time in front of the principal's office. And when an outbreak occurred, fever and bleeding and pain, he withdrew into such interesting activities—his stamps, his trains, his independent-study programs—that it was quite a long time before I became aware of the amount of solitude he bore.

In the same way did the physical changes sneak up on us. Sam had been sick for some eight months by the spring of 1963. During that period the time spans between acute episodes of the disease, called exacerbations, became shorter and shorter, and it seemed to me that he was in almost constant pain, though sometimes that was difficult to ascertain because he didn't own up to pain; it was a matter of observing the spasms in his belly as they were mirrored on his face.

Then, on a lovely day in April, looking out the window and seeing Sam and Tom from across the street standing under the crabapple tree which was raining down pink petals on them, I became aware that something was odd. What? And suddenly knew. Sam had always been taller than Tom; now they were the same size. When Sam came inside, I said to him that Tommy had certainly shot up lately. He gave me a look that might have been ironic. "Yeah," he agreed, "and so have all the kids in my class. I used to be second tallest after Robert."

"Oh, well, Robert! He's giant," I replied nervously, afraid to find out what Sam had meant.

The next time we saw Dr. Freeman, I watched closely as he measured and weighed Sam. And later spoke to him on the telephone. He confirmed that Sam had not grown during the last year, that he was down to sixty-five pounds. "But he weighed eighty-five last summer!" I protested.

"Yes." Dr. Freeman cleared his throat, then he said gently that I knew—"Don't you, Jean?"—that retardation of growth was one of the complications of the disease. Yes, I said, and hung up, again terribly aware of my helplessness, and the uncertainty. I mean, what were we doing? It wasn't that I didn't trust Dr. Freeman—he was always a comfort with his warmth and availability. He wasn't like Dr. Burns, who, on being told that we had consulted a specialist, reportedly said, "Good! I hate treating ulcerative colitis." No, Dr. Freeman cared, and he consulted regularly with the specialist.

But was that enough? All our inquiries had confirmed that the nice, simple man in New Haven was indeed an authority. Mark and I joked about it, calling him the "Maven from Yale" and the "Genius from Connecticut"—all of which probably expressed our unease. Why didn't he *do* something?

Walking away from the telephone, I thought of all that. Mark was off on one of his business trips, about which I was having ambivalent feelings. On one hand, I hated to be left alone with all the problems, and yet I wanted Mark to go, so he could keep exploring other medical systems—the milk-free diet in Britain, the psychiatric approach in a Swiss sanitarium—something, anything, just so that we weren't standing still at the bottom of the hill while the truck came rushing down at us. Out of control.

Speaking of ambivalence, Sam's illness was changing all our perceptions. I suppose until that time, Mark and I had indulged in the usual arrogance of the healthy. We had had only one previous encounter with real vulnerability—when Papa died, and we had found ourselves so profoundly bereft. Mark had always enjoyed his extraordinary relationship with his father, loving and close; I think Papa was the last of the great listeners. When Mark and I married I became part of their union, which gave my life a completely new dimension. As far as I was concerned, I simply hadn't had enough of this when Papa died before he was sixty. Still, after a while, we had come to terms with acceptance and adulthood and being next in line, the whole syndrome of loss. After which we had, I think, blossomed into a kind of pride of survival.

Just because the pain had been so bad, was it extra sweet to have mastered it? I don't really know. Certainly, we had not consciously dwelt on our ability to have overcome. Yet I think now that we felt that it was our personal worth, our fine psychological tuning, our lovely genes—I mean, all three children had my blond hair—as well as other factors in our control, which were responsible for our good fortune. Look at us: these marvelous kids, growing financial security, and all that love in our house!

Then this chaos. And didn't it follow that if we took credit for our enviable status, we now had to assume the guilt for the misfortune? What had we done to our Sam? Nor was our situation made easier by public ignorance about the disease and the almost universal assumption that anything with the word "colitis" attached to it must be psychosomatic. Sam, I was told repeatedly by our friends, was the "type," of course. Yes, of course: so earnest, so inner, and always getting good marks in school. And weren't we the perfect example of compulsive parents? Look at the way Mark worked, on top of being president of the synagogue. And I, handling the cultural program and being president of the Israel Bonds drive. And my writing. And look at the house I ran. And Daniel at Brandeis! All achievers, achievers. The new dirty word.

At the same time that we felt guilty, we were angry. Not only at the doctors who didn't help, or at our friends who talked nonsense. No, also angry at each other. For instance, I hated the look of concern with which Mark came home each night and his saying, "How is he?" first thing. And we constantly argued physical protection vs. psychological consideration; Mark said I was obsessed with my determination that Sam wasn't to be made to feel different. He said that it was madness to have permitted him to go on a certain bike trip, that Sam was a sensible kid who could understand perfectly well that he needed extra rest to fight off the exacerbation. No, I came back, no. Sam needed large doses of reassurance that he was still himself; it was worth taking chances. But while we were all trying to do the "right," the "good" thing, we also had to cope with our annoyance at Sam, who refused to improve as a result of all our care. Maybe Rachel told the story best. She was seven; her teacher gave her an A and marked the paper "Delightful."

Once there was a bad bunny. He always did what he was not supposed to do. He ran in fields and went in a bucket of water. And he lost his new shoes. When he went in the bucket he got a cold. When he got home he had to go to bed. And he had soup for supper. His name is Sam.

The others had cookies and cherries. But Sam had his mother tell him a story.

So there it was, with the accusation built in. If he had only stayed out of the bucket of water! It served him right that he couldn't have cookies and cherries. But damn it, he did get his mother to sit at his bed and tell him a story.

When summer came around, I refused to go back to Hampton Bays. I came on strong; I thought my reasoning was sound. Look, I said to Mark, it would be bad for all of us to return to the scene of the crime. God, just thinking of the place made me smell Lysol. Think how much worse it must be for Sam, who had suffered so atrociously in that place. What we needed, I told all of them, was a change of pace, something new, different, exciting. Daniel shrugged; he was going back to Israel for the summer. Mark finally agreed, though reluctantly. But Rachel was enthusiastic.

As to Sam, he kept repeating that we *always* go to Hampton Bays, why not this year? I suppressed mentioning that he also hated to buy new shoes because he didn't like to part from his old ones, and that this whole "always" business was ridiculous in a kid. Instead I argued reasonably, "Don't you want to go mountain climbing and explore caves? And maybe Daddy will take you on that little train up to the top of Mount Washington." I spread out the alluring brochure, showing him the fairy-tale red train chugging steeply upward through luscious green toward a white peak.

"Can I go, can I go?" Rachel shouted, but I used bribery to elicit Sam's enthusiasm and told Rachel that no, this was an outing for the boys; they said that it got very cold up on the mountain. Which made Sam agree that it might be fun.

Oh, nightmare New Hampshire! Dreadful Bretton Woods, torturous hikes in that most grandiose landscape, along narrow pine-needle-carpeted paths, under towering trees, playing Indian with determination against all odds because ten, twelve, fourteen times there had to be the rush to relieve the cramps. A broad, shallow brook to ford, schools of tiny fish flashing brilliantly between feet planted on separate flat stones; Rachel sitting contentedly catching polliwogs in her Mason jar with the lid riddled with holes. Rachel round in her leopard-printed tank suit, and Sam all ribs with his trunks barely hanging on bony hips: both of them poised to dive off the stone ledge into the deep pool under the waterfall. Mark already in the icy water yelling, Come on, come on, and I, as usual: Be careful! And then seeing the three of them below me and watching Rachel, the seal, bursting with joy and Mark caught in his water madness, but Sam searching the steep rocks all around for a place to scramble out, panic in his eyes. Reaching a hand to him, pulling him up. "Are you okay, Sam?" "Sure, fine." And he was off into the woods.

The worst, maybe, was the meals. Two bites, perhaps three, and then the look. And watching him trying to fight it down, but finally saying, "Can I be excused?" and giving Mark a disdainful look when he asked to come along. "Why does Sam have to throw up all the time?" Rachel would ask, and I would say, "Don't talk with your mouth full" and try to go on eating. And Mark would ask, "How was the tennis?" Rachel was taking lessons; the pro said she was amazingly apt.

One day Rachel went off on an outing with a children's group and we took Sam horseback riding. On a trail that was like the aisle in a high-domed church with sun rays breaking through greens and golds of stained glass, with only the sound of an unseen stream rushing nearby. Single file: Mark, Sam, I. And suddenly the tears were streaming down my cheeks as I saw the narrow back in front of me, a small stick figure, dwarfed yet more by the broadness of the horse's back. Something made Sam's horse shy at that moment, and he came sailing off the rump and landed in moss. He laughed and laughed. In a flash we were next to him. He looked at me, surprised. "Why are you crying, Mom?"

"Are you hurt?"

" 'Course not." And scrambled back on to the high perch.

That night I gave in. "Okay, it's ridiculous; let's go home."

Luckily, our house in Hampton Bays was still available. The day before we left New Hampshire, Mark and Sam took the train up Mt. Washington, but Sam had to remain in the hut at the top because it was too bitterly cold. When we were alone, Mark said that Rachel would have been able to tolerate it better up there. I searched his face, trying to know what he was saying. Was he angry, ironic, sad? All three. And more.

MARCH 5, 1977

I had not had a tachycardia like this in years. And while Sam and Mark had dinner downstairs, upstairs I walked back and forth, back and forth, waiting for the magic combination of Librium and phenobarb to stop the crazy feeling that I had a racing motor inside me. Like riding a bike, it is apparently unforgettable how to behave in a state of acute anxiety. I knew that lying down would be bad, that I would feel as if the force of my heartbeat were shaking the bed, which would scare me even more; so I paced. When it got a bit better, I perched on the edge of the bed and tried to do last Sunday's unfinished puzzle.

It was almost comical the way it was coming back to me how to handle this situation effectively, the way I remembered that reading would be impossible but that the crossword puzzle, with its demand for short-span concentration—one word at a time—would fill the bill and distract me from the panic. Mark came upstairs a couple of times to ask whether I was all right, and the first time I could only nod and motion him away, but the next time I said that I was almost out of it and for him to relax. Finally, I was able to crawl under the covers, and when Mark came to bed I held close to him. So the night passed, snatches of sleep, each terminated when the sledgehammer of full consciousness would whang us awake, but toward morning I did fall into a real sleep and was roused only by the awaited telephone call from Rachel's morning nurse.

We had met her a few days earlier; she was in to see Rachel several times, and introduced her to other patients who had undergone the same surgery. At one time there was a gathering of six "pouchies" at the bedside of a girl just four days postop. The others were from two to six weeks after their surgery. Rachel had seemed less overwhelmed by this than I felt, and she had also accepted the prevalent humor, the nickname "pouchy," the reference to "kangeroo power."

Of course, if you accept the premise that the more you know the better off you are, which is Rachel's firm conviction, then all this was a very reassuring experience. In any case, meeting both her morning and her afternoon nurses in advance was helpful to all of us. Additionally we were told that these women were Dr. Gaon's best nurses, that they had been specially trained for this procedure; and Rachel liked them both. Personally I was more impressed with the morning nurse, who was brash, cheerful, and positive, though both Rachel and Mark were more sensitively predicting that the other one would wear better.

Anyhow, this morning the voice of Norma Berliner was a hosannah from above. "All systems go!" she proclaimed, and said that Rachel was doing splendidly; they were waiting for an orderly to wheel them back from the recovery room to Klingenstein, and she would administer a big shot of morphine the minute they got into Rachel's room. "I see no reason for Rach' to be in pain," she said. I hung up in a glow; repeated everything to Mark, who'd appeared, wrapped in a towel, out of the shower, and to Sam who was also suddenly there. "All systems go!" We all laughed. Underneath, I was aware of the implication of the talk of the morphine and that my question about the degree of Rachel's pain had not so much been swept away as drowned in Norma's chatter.

But when we finally walk into Rachel's room, she is so much herself that I am buoyed by a swell of relief. She wants to talk, to tell us about the nightmare of the recovery room and about the awful nurse who, after getting permission to medicate Rachel every three hours, had withheld punctual administration of the morphine while she had a long private telephone conversation. "I couldn't believe it, Mom. I thought I knew something about pain, but this . . . I kept calling the nurse, please, please, but she just went on and on." Rachel closes her eyes; I feel consumed with hatred for the faceless woman in the recovery room.

Then Rachel explains the function of the N.G. (nasal gastric) tube which runs from her stomach, through her nose, into a machine which keeps pumping out her stomach juices. It flashes red each time it starts up. We see brown-red liquid come bubbling out of Rachel's nose and travel along the clear plastic tubing into the large glass jar at the bottom of the machine. I try to keep my eyes off it as Rachel speaks of the Foley catheter, the catheter that leads from her bladder into an output bag attached to the bed. She boasts that Norma says her output is sensational, and then she points to the several I.V. bottles—antibiotic, albumin, steroid, glucose. Attempting to take the situation in, I keep listening for the voice behind the educated reporter, behind that distant onlooker in this room of strange odors—not bad, not disgusting: just strange.

And all the time we are under the patter of a steady rain—the voice of Norma the nurse, who, after a short positive account of Rachel's condition, is also telling us about her boyfriend, her tennis game, and what she's going to cook for her dinner party that night. Also that this actor on the soap opera she watches, who's married to this woman on the show, has actually divorced his real-life wife, with whom he has five children, in order to wed the one he's married to on the show. "Isn't that super?" she asks me. "So romantic." I look at her, expecting a grin, a sign that she's kidding, but no, her open face is enthusiastic; and all the time she is turning Rachel deftly, doing things efficiently, with a sure hand.

Now Rachel's face is very white. "My back is the worst of it," she says, and Norma wedges a pillow firmly against it and talks on. I seem to be the main target; somehow I respond as if I were at a tea party, listening politely, trying to seem interested. In the meantime, Mark is holding Rachel's hand and Sam is talking quietly to her; but then Sam turns to Norma and interrupts the deluge to ask when Rachel is due for the next shot. Norma nods and agrees that it's time, yeah, a little earlier won't hurt, she'll square it with the doctor later, she'll be right back. At last we are alone and suddenly, all of us, without words. Rachel closes her eyes. She looks very frail and very beautiful. Crazily, the contrast puts me in mind of the Rachel she was that summer in New Hampshire.

✿　✿　✿

Hampton Bays turned out to be better. Not that Sam was less ill; it was just that there were fewer demands on him or us—no formal meals among strangers, no historic sites to compel sight-seeing. We all relaxed on the better days and somehow bore up on the bad ones. But even the good days always started badly; invariably I awoke to the running footsteps, and by the time I saw Sam he'd have dark rings under his eyes, hair stuck to his forehead, the signs of ordeal. Sometimes this morning siege took a few hours, but mostly he began to feel better by ten or eleven. Then we actually went to the beach, and he dived into the breakers, and my fears were multiplied endlessly; he was so light, like a bobbing piece of driftwood in the force of the turmoiled ocean. I prayed for calm waters.

Prayed for calm waters. A symbolic phrase? Or did I actually pray in those days? Certainly I remember being ambivalent about prayer even then. I think I was more inclined toward thankfulness than toward making demands of God. Probably I was too afraid of my rage. The rest of the family did not share my attitude. Mark was very big on religion; I'd watch him in synagogue, see the intensity of his involvement in the prayers and feel an alienation like a summer breeze—light, quick. It was so strange to me when I knew that actually, really, if I made him face it, look at it, question it, he "believed" no more than I. Yet I felt that these were mean thoughts, because, what did it matter as long as it helped him? Why insist on rationalism?

As a matter of fact, it was I who had seriously brought God into the picture for Sam. It was during a terrible exacerbation when Sam sort of lost hold of his usual pose and asked the big why's. Why me, why so bad, why? And all that came to me was that I didn't know, but that perhaps God had something special in mind for him. Sam thought that over and then said, nodding, "Like, to make me tough?" Scared, I nodded back. Oh, I was a fine one to insist on rational thought. In any case, it worked for Sam too. I'd see him put his hand on his head in fulfillment of the commandment that an Orthodox Jew's head be covered before God. The gesture—his hand a makeshift *yarmulke*, or prayer cap—became a familiar one. He prayed at odd moments I couldn't fathom. Later the gesture became abbreviated to a fleeting touch of his head whenever he was anxious. It was also clear that going to synagogue was meaningful to Sam, whether exclusively for prayer or because it provided a special togetherness with Mark.

Rachel apparently caught my ambivalences. She said synagogue was okay, but she slept through the rabbi's sermons. Or perhaps she sensed how much I enjoyed shifting the sleeping child more ostentatiously into the hollow of my arm, smiling apologetically at the rabbi or at anyone else who happened to notice us.

Why the spite? I had a crutch too. A long analysis, begun after Papa died and I was afflicted with the bouts of tachycardia and my sense of vulnerability. While this analysis was doing some very good things for me—liberating, supporting, and providing insights —it never progressed to the recognition of my terrible anger. Rage, I guess, at our present situation too. Which might have been the reason why, right after the summer, I began to suggest that Sam see a child psychiatrist. Perhaps I thought that Sam might succeed in dealing with this rage I felt might devour him, and I was impressed with the idea of what the doctors called supportive therapy. The very term seemed to express exactly what Sam needed: therapy, equaling treatment of disease, and supportive, to help him. Because I couldn't.

Of course, he wouldn't hear of it; he was full of preconceived notions. A boy in his class was known to go to a shrink and apparently quoted him a lot. In all fairness, if the child was to be believed, that psychiatrist said some very peculiar things. I countered Sam's argument by reminding him that Ralph Berk was also a psychiatrist and did he think that Ralph was weird or that it would be hard to talk to him? No. And okay, he would speak to Ralph. Then the explanation that psychiatrists do not treat friends. "But treat, how?" Sam asked. "For what? I am not crazy."

"Of course not. But it's helpful to talk to someone who understands."

"You understand. Dad does."

"Yes. But we are too close to you."

Sam was adjusting a switch on his railroad when we had this conversation. It was fall; he had been out of school for a week already. He looked up at me, asked, "You mean it hurts you too much?"

My face burning, I met his eyes, said, "Yes." Then, when he didn't answer me, I felt the heat spread down, into my neck and shoulders, and was scared that I had said the wrong thing, that Mark would be furious, that Sam would know . . . know what? What was wrong with what I had said? It was right to be straight with Sam; how else would he ever trust me again? I went on, speaking quickly, "And a psychiatrist can help you to understand the anger you feel at us too."

"Why should I be angry at you?" He was coupling the milk train to the log carrier.

"Because we can't make it go away."

Sam started his engine fast—too fast. He watched it career down the track and crash at the next curve. He jumped up, kicked the station house, yelled, "Dumb! Stupid, dumb toy."

In the end he went, of course. Did he have a choice? We were scrupulous not to pressure him, but the weight of my anxiety must have been too much. And perhaps he was not yet convinced of our impotence—he might have thought that there must be merit in something I championed. Though first he made very damn sure that his father shared my views.

It was a day in November, cold, blowy; the three of us, Mark, Sam, and I, went for the first appointment together. In the doctor's office the radiator hissed, and he had all of us talking; we found the hour short. Afterward, on the way home, we laughed quite a lot; the doctor had been jolly, though none of us could recall what he looked like. I asked Sam the following week, when he came downstairs after seeing the doctor by himself, whether he had noted his looks on that visit. Sam said no, but boy, Dr. Chevalier knew about stamps; he had a brand-new Scott's catalog, the '64 edition, and next time he'd show Sam his Egyptian first-day covers.

Finally, Mark and I went alone. For an evaluation. Oh, I was very tight, already defiant; don't let him come at me with any of his psychiatric crap! Looking at him, I at last saw the scar on his forehead—accident, smash, suffering, pain—also warmth, niceness. "That kid needs a psychiatrist like a hole in the head," Dr. Chevalier said first off. "I can't think how anyone else could handle this rotten situation any better."

Suddenly I could breathe again, saw Mark sit back, take out his pipe. A person. The doctor was a person. He liked Sam. We could talk to him. We decided that just the same, it would be a good idea for the doctor to build a relationship with Sam. "Be Dr. Chevalier, his knight, his friend," Dr. Chevalier said, and I did not think that the concept was corny. "He'll need someone to trust aside from his parents when the time comes . . ." which was when I turned the juice off again. The time wouldn't come; something would happen. Suddenly I was telling him about my therapy, the way I had experienced symptom relief almost immediately, that I hadn't had a tachycardia in years. I talked fast until I became aware of the eyes of the doctor on me and felt that Mark was also watching me. Then I stopped. No. "No," I said, "I guess this is a different situation." Dr. Chevalier nodded.

So I began to drive Sam to New York to see Dr. Chevalier once a week. They played stamps. Only Sam objected to the word "played." They traded, sorted, worked on the stamps.

"And what else?" I asked.

"What do you mean: what else?"

"Don't you talk?"

"Sure we talk."

I knew better, but it was hard to shut up, not to ask. However, Sam made it easier by ignoring my probing. As usual, he had the right instinct about appropriate behavior. He was not to be invaded.

During the next year Dr. Chevalier taught Sam to curse, to defy his father on the issue of changing out of wet swim trunks on hot days; and he acquainted him with the idea that he had a deadly disease. While Sam had his sessions, I used to wait for him in the car. With my note pad on my knee, scribbling furiously; I had burst into a rage of poetry. It was one of the things my analysis had re-uncovered, this need to write, dormant since adolescence. And one day, when Sam came out, he settled himself into his seat, turned to look at me, and said, "Did you know that one can die from ulcerative colitis?"

My head snapped up. I too had been dealing with death. But in an abstract way, iambic; most of all: intellectually.

Sam repeated, "People die from ulcerative colitis."

"Not many," I said, and cut a funny face. Like, Oh, well! But inside, I felt a storm of protest, and all the good feeling for Dr. Chevalier went out the window. What the hell was he doing? And why?

Sam insisted, "Yes, many." He quoted statistics; thirty-one percent.

In the meantime, we had learned a great deal about ulcerative colitis. I would even say that Mark and I knew considerably more about it than the average doctor. In fact, it was amazing to us how much ignorance the doctors of our acquaintance expressed, the impossible diets urged upon us, the always recurring theme of "nerves." One Ear Nose and Throat man whom we met at a cocktail party declared that children with ulcerative colitis did best when removed from their parents. Luckily, we were already pretty well informed by the time we met him, so I could reply politely that I knew of the failure of that particular experiment, and at what hospital it had been conducted, and that the young patients who had been paired in a one-to-one relationship with psychiatrists had not really improved. "On the other hand," I said with what I thought was a pleasant smile, "I understand that the participating psychiatrists suffered much damage." Dr. Ear Nose and Throat looked insulted and moved to another group of drinkers. There he raised his voice sufficiently to let me hear that he thought it sad that parents of sick children had so much need to deny. I laughed, but it hurt.

Everything hurt. Hurt like hell. Learning about doctors' egos, learning that they weren't the kindly, all-powerful giants of our childhood perceptions, learning that it made them angry and mean when they had to deal with something they didn't understand: all that hurt. So I didn't get too excited when our cousin Gustav, who was a dermatologist, called one day and said that he wanted us to see a young gastroenterologist whose article he had just read in the *New York State Journal of Medicine*.

Gustav had been very supportive throughout, the one person with whom we could really consult. We had filtered all our information through him; he had checked out countless names, rumors, and drugs for us. But the most important thing was that he was always honest and unpretentious. He could actually say that he didn't know something. And he cared; he was as scared as we were about the way Sam was going down.

I said sure, we'd read the article, but in any case we'd first see this doctor without Sam. We had done that several times in order to spare Sam the ordeal of repeated x-rays; examinations; most of all, personalities. Many of those visits had proven senseless; by now we understood that the pool of existing knowledge was simply not very deep. Gustav agreed, but he made it clear that he did not want us to procrastinate on this one, and something in the way he said it made me suddenly feel very excited. When Mark came home I infected him with my urgency. "Let's go down now; Gustl sounded insistent. Let's borrow his copy of the article."

However, when we got there, while Gustav and his wife, Bella, had brewed fresh coffee and were serving hot coffee cake, Gustl only handed us a torn-out page from the journal. One look at an out-of-context sentence at the top of it and at the next line in heavy print—PROGRAM OF MANAGEMENT, obviously a new subheading—made it clear that our cousin was not showing us the complete article. There were various reasons he cited: ". . . the rest is purely technical; you wouldn't understand it anyhow." And ". . . I do need the journal tonight; I'm preparing a paper myself." References, biographies, etcetera. We argued. At last, angrily, he agreed to let us read it, but we were not to take it home.

Then Mark and I sat next to each other on the couch in the consultation room, suddenly alone, suddenly scared, no longer certain why we had insisted. And tried to read. It seemed to me that Mark was quite businesslike about it; he was taking notes. But he had to wait for me to turn the pages, because I had a most difficult time focusing, not to mention concentrating.

The article started innocently enough with the statement that ten to fifteen percent of all patients with ulcerative colitis get ill before their sixteenth birthday. Then it went on to describe typical symptoms that may occur at the onset of the disease, and it said that children are subject to all the known ravages and complications such as urgency, bloody diarrhea, cramps, pain, debilitation and dehydration, neuralgia, arthritis . . . Then followed some words which, on consultation, neither of us understood, though we deduced one to concern a skin condition, the other some kind of toxemia; and then it spoke of perforations, hemorrhages, fistulas, abscesses, eye disease, and depression. Increasingly nauseated, I said loudly that Sam wasn't the least bit depressed, nor did he have *all* the symptoms they were describing. But was struck dumb by the next sentence which began: "Potentially irreversible retardation of growth and development . . ."

After that I read in a haze except for the sharp attention I gave to a diagram on the second page. It almost looked like a family tree. Underneath, the caption stated that it represented the prognosis of eighty-four children with ulcerative colitis. And there it was—in percentages yet: those who would live, those who would develop carcinoma, have ileostomies, be "deceased" (Sam's "31%"); I raged at the obscene word.

Then I skimmed, a sentence here and there. "55% required definitive surgery." "Food per se, does not appear to be an etiologic factor except perhaps for milk . . ." (Oh, the British study!) And the mention of Azulfidine, a drug Sam had lately been given. ". . . many reports of favorable influence [but] the over-all results are not impressive." By the time the discussion in the paper progressed into the use of hormonal therapy, I was all at once too fatigued to go on. I rose, leaving Mark to it.

Back in the living room, Bella poured more coffee, talked in her warm, quick voice. Gustav glowered, then exploded. "This was necessary? You had to read it? So! And did it enlighten you? Are you feeling good?" Bella told him to leave me alone. I said, punch-drunk, that it was okay, I hadn't taken it in anyhow. I actually laughed. "Would you believe it? I've known about the possibility of surgery from the beginning, but I keep forgetting. And I still don't know what an ileostomy is. No, don't tell me!" My voice shrill: I heard it up there; loud, not at all like mine. I added,

"Every time I hear it mentioned it's a surprise." Then I was quiet, looking down on my hands, how elegantly I was holding my cup; my fingers didn't even tremble; I was in control. And Bella's voice, a pleasant rill. Then Mark, white-faced, stowing a whole lot of notes into his breast pocket, saying, "Come on, let's let Gustl and Bella go to sleep." He picked up the page that we were to take home, he thanked them for coffee and cake, he steered me out.

In the car, driving, I realized that I knew every word on the pages I had read. I could see the exact way in which the article had been set up: the title, ULCERATIVE COLITIS IN CHILDREN; the doctor's name, also in block letters, though smaller. Mark reached for my hand, squeezed it. And when we were almost at home, he said, "Tomorrow, when we're calmer, we'll study this 'program of management'—okay?" I nodded, certain that Mark would know that I agreed. Though I could not talk just then.

CHAPTER 3

JUNE 7, 1965

After Four Days

Tonight I left
after these eons of vigil;
I left him with the friendly nurse
so brisk, so quick, so white . . .
and I step abroad into moonlight
and stars and healthy people.
Prepared to be split into fragments
of here-and-thereness,
in guilty delight at my escape
but deeply aware
of the pieces of me in chain
. . .
and he can not fly forth.

MARCH 6, 1977

Uncannily the same, yet so different. Perhaps because in some ways, to myself at least, I was the star, the interesting one in the sense in which an adult with her greater range of perceptions is more interesting than a child. Of course, it is not that way with Rachel. She is in control even as she needs to be turned and held and ministered to; it is we who are the bit players, who are told when she wants a glycerin lemon swab for her dry lips. It reminds me of another poem I wrote during Sam's illness. I had called it "Let Not My Pity Be His Trap."

No question of pity now. A kind of fury to see Rachel suffer. And while I can feel the business of the here-and-thereness again and the guilt at the relief each time I leave, there is no thought of being split into fragments. Rachel's wholeness leaves me whole. I suppose it is the difference between the symbiosis of the mother–child relationship and the equality between consenting adults. Temporarily, Rachel is consenting to let me fill her needs, though always with her finger raised in admonition: don't trespass, don't presume; most of all, don't take over. Which makes it both harder and easier than it was with Sam.

"Who of Dad's admirers sent this one?" Rachel asks when another huge flower arrangement arrives. The joke is wearing thin; Mark's business acquaintances are being very kind. "To think that I'll have to write all those thank-you notes!" she wails. I tell her to stop complaining; say, "Look at those gorgeous spring flowers!" Outside, the park is white in snow. Together we try to name them: daffodils, tulips, forsythia, larkspur, delphiniums . . . "Yes, nice," she admits. "Put them on the windowsill where I can see them. The room looks like an arboretum."

Everyone says that Rachel is doing splendidly. Yesterday she made two telephone calls. She wants to talk of the recovery room, to tell me how it was—the feeling of being caught, an animal in a trap, the pain tearing her into ragged pieces. "And the noise!" She puts her hands over her ears, winces as the quick movement tugs at the I.V. in her left hand. "But most of all the helplessness," she says, "the incredible helplessness against the pain." Her words trail off, she closes her eyes, a tear squeezes past. I stroke her face, say, "Don't think of it," but I know she will.

Yes, today is not great. The surgeon has readjusted the tube in her pouch which had caused her discomfort, and the backache is still excruciating. Nanette Sheffler, the pixieish afternoon nurse, is rubbing her back patiently. Otherwise, Rachel has a rash and she itches; they are talking of discontinuing the antibiotic to which she might be allergic. "Isn't it too soon?" I worry.

"I have no fever," she explains in the hoarse voice the tube in her throat is giving her.

I feel very upset. What have you done for me lately, God? I have already taken it for granted that all has gone well, feel outraged at her pain, shocked that she awaits the morphine so eagerly, afraid of later when she will have to walk again. Day Two. Though they had her doing it yesterday already. Relentlessly. And what did I expect?

❧ ❧ ❧

When we went to see Dr. Paul Zalinger, the author of the article Gustl had let us read, we took Sam with us after all. We had assimilated the ideas behind his suggested management already; to our minds it was innovative and daring as well as conservative and safe. A long telephone discussion with Gustav bore out that we understood it correctly. I had called him to apologize for our insistence on reading the paper; he had countered by saying that he was sorry to have yelled at me. A minuet, because we were fond of each other. But really we both knew that, right or wrong, Mark and I were forever altered by the experience of reading that paper.

I kept thinking of a childhood fairy tale about a girl who had been told that she might never enter a certain room. I could no longer remember the details or even the point or the outcome of the story, only the fact that curiosity persuaded her to disobey. Inside the forbidden room she touched a golden spinning wheel and later found that the gold on her finger would not wash off. That is how I felt—that we were marked. Yet we tried to wriggle out from under our new knowledge. Mark, in spite of his business-like notes, was even more adept than I. He had obviously put his effort into the "writing down" rather than the "taking in." So it was a struggle to understand the method of management discussed, but at last we had.

Simply put, the proposal was to try hormonal therapy in children who had not responded to conservative treatment. Apparently fairly large dosages were involved, and if they produced good response the steroids should be reduced very gradually and maintained at low levels until clinical appearance of the colon was normal. Then, if symptoms recurred, the medication should be increased or restarted, and later again reduced but still more slowly. If all this were to fail, the article stated, surgery should be considered. Of course surgery would be urgent if there were perforations or massive bleeding or cancer or strictures or abscesses, but it would be elective if after two years of therapy there were still smoldering symptoms of the primary disease, etcetera, etcetera.

The question I had not been able to bring myself to ask Gustav concerned a sentence that kept running through my mind. It stated that the program gave the child the reasonable opportunity to respond to a medical program ". . . even at the sacrifice of developing a bizarre and even grotesque appearance." It further explained that most parents were willing to tolerate and even enthusiastically accept these circumstances when reassured of their reversibility and because the program offered a chance of avoiding the radical surgery—a total proctocolectomy (removal of colon and rectum), which was the only other known cure for ulcerative colitis.

On the way to Dr. Zalinger's office my primary anxiety revolved around this mystery—bizarre and even grotesque, how? I realized that Mark and I completely avoided discussing what this meant. We concentrated on the positive aspect—that this doctor was willing to "do something," not sit by passively with the attitude that the case either would come to surgery or not. No, he had devised a program that gave a "reasonable opportunity to respond." And since 1958, out of twenty children with ulcerative colitis who had been managed according to the principles of this program, only three had been medical failures requiring surgery.

He was tall, slim, silver gray. The youthful face was edged with deep lines along the cheeks. His handshake was firm, his voice was resonant; he was young-old. Only the fact that there was moisture on his forehead provided proof of his . . . well, what? Humanity? In contrast to being godlike? I kept telling myself that it was our expectations that endowed him with so much extraordinary power, our needs, our wishes, our hopes. And our fears. Regardless, he was larger than life. When Sam went off with him to be examined after we had the preliminary conversation, something in the way Sam looked up at him, laughed with him, and then, from the adjoining examining room, the way their voices mingled, though we couldn't hear what they said, made me feel relieved, as if we had reached safe harbor. Looking at Mark, I knew that he was also satisfied.

Later all three of us sat facing Dr. Zalinger's desk. He addressed himself mostly to Sam, explaining his program to him. Sam was rapt. I watched him, the old pride in his perfectness surfacing, his fine face, intelligent brow, the questions he asked; Dr. Zalinger answered them seriously. And there it was, though more nicely put, ". . . your face will moon; you will look quite fat," the doctor said, explaining the effect the steroids would have. Sam shrugged:

so what, as long as he would regain his appetite, the weight he had lost, have no more bleeding or pain.

I wanted, desperately, to share Sam's confidence, wanted to forget about bizarre and even grotesque. To look fat and have a moon face wasn't so bad, and anyhow, it was impossible to picture Sam looking like that. I thought back to the steroids he had taken at Presbyterian Hospital. Could there be all that much difference between fifteen and sixty milligrams?

After a while Dr. Zalinger asked Sam to step out for a little while. "Do you mind? I'd like to talk to your parents alone now." Sam nodded, got up; I could see that something in the straightforward way in which he was being treated made him want to cooperate. However, Mark and I could actually only repeat the questions Sam had already asked, though I did bring up "grotesque." Dr. Zalinger said it would not be for long. He used the phrase "completely reversible," and it occurred to me only when we were driving home that he never mentioned the possibility of surgical intervention; we were set on a course to succeed. God, Dr. Zalinger was positive!

Sam was crazy about him—an affection that lasted through the weekly office visits, which must have been fairly uncomfortable. It was the more remarkable because Sam, like Mark, was a cautious type when it came to making friends. Of course, there was the dramatic cessation of symptoms, which swung all of us high into the air—no more pain, urgency, diarrhea, and Sam was enjoying his food again. But even when the unpleasant side effects of the steroids hit, when the weight gain we had welcomed so enthusiastically kept mounting and mounting and Sam would be breathless with a racing inner motor and his joints hurt him, even then he remained loyal in his complete confidence that Dr. Zalinger would turn this thing around.

And basically Mark shared Sam's feeling. Here were two men—calling each other Mark and Paul almost immediately—close in age, high in accomplishments, and it was as if the boy in each was making quick contact with the other, a rapprochement. Mark would bring a Havana or two home from overseas business trips and share them with the doctor; Sam was the willing delivery boy. And he took the twelve little white pills—sixty milligrams of Prednisone—each day and then rejoiced when the dose was reduced to eleven.

My feelings were much more complex. I too would fall under

the spell of the doctor's confidence, his warmth, his vitality, when I sat across from him. But away from his presence I questioned some of the things he said, his peculiar humor especially. And I was disturbed by the fact that it appeared to me that he had joined our conspiracy of denial; it was as if he as well kept forgetting that the possibility of surgery existed. Mark, with whom I discussed these misgivings, said that was ridiculous, that Paul knew what he was doing. ". . . look, when I go to a customer, I expect to sell," Mark elaborated. "I don't talk about, or even think of, the possibility that he has too large an inventory!"

"Okay, exactly!" I shot back. "That's what I mean—perhaps Dr. Zalinger uses too much salesmanship; we are not dealing with a product here."

"Yes, we are. He has to believe in his method of management in exactly the way I have to believe in my product." Then, a little angrily, "It's this romance you make of doctors and rabbis! Expecting them to be God."

Not God, I thought, but special. Better, maybe, like good fathers. I shut up; Mark had a point, and since I was just then terminating my analysis, I knew I'd have to watch against bringing to Dr. Zalinger the set of complicated emotions with which I was still saddled.

Way into Sam's second year of illness, it was Christmas again and we went to Puerto Rico that winter. Sam was now a small boy whose swollen legs were striated in inflamed streaks. His belly was inflated and taut, his neck had practically disappeared between the fat shoulders, and he had pouched cheeks which were always a shiny red. Oh, looking grotesque, all right. But we were on the way down off the steroids, down to twenty milligrams, only four pills. Soon the reversal of these secondary symptoms would occur and Sam would reemerge, himself, but without acute ulcerative colitis. He would go back to school, strange kids would no longer call him Blimp or Fatso, he would take the Ace bandages off his poor legs, would no longer waddle, would be swift and beautiful and well.

We all believed that fervently, intensely, which was what made that vacation bearable. The expectation of return out of the cruel metamorphosis had Sam already swimming in the blue-green ocean, had him disregarding the pain in his legs, hitting tennis balls, and even being less self-conscious in public. It was almost behind him.

We had a beachfront cottage, and at night I would lie and look into the floodlit palms, at the shining rocks, and into the confectionary-sugar spray of the moonlit breakers, and I would know that there was also a great deal of prayer in our good expectations. Except that none of us dared to be that tentative. In fact, Mark and I did a lot of arguing about our attitude toward religion during that time. I think I was trying to say to him that he could do without the superstitious rituals, that all would be well.

Until a morning two days before we were to fly home when I saw Sam, on leaving the dining room, prepare himself for the five-minute walk back to our rooms by putting his hand on his head. I saw his lips moving before he started off; he was praying to make it. And knew what that meant. Later in the day he told me that he was bleeding again. On the telephone, Dr. Zalinger said to resume sixty milligrams of Prednisone. "Mark," he said—I was listening in on the extension—"Mark, I know how you feel! But I'll get him off it again as soon as possible."

That was a very bad year. We learned a new language. Sam "escaped" each time he was down to fifteen or twenty milligrams of the Prednisone, had "exacerbations," swung between the primary symptoms of the disease and the secondary ones caused by the steroids. School was a constant problem, and it was finally I who discouraged him from going after I began to understand the additional terror school was imposing on him: the concern about his appearance and, more unbearable, about his dignity—perhaps about his life. Was that why Dr. Chevalier had brought the issue into the open? To let Sam talk about it? In any case, once the decision was made for him to stay home for a while, he seemed somewhat easier.

We settled into a routine built around seeing the doctors. I tried to imbue these excursions with the aura of being a treat, tried to countermand the depression Sam could not verbalize except by criticizing the air and filth in the streets of New York. Really violently, as we crossed the George Washington Bridge, "I hate New York!" So we studied the Lionel catalog before each trip and decided which piece of railroad equipment Sam needed, and while sometimes it was only a length of special wire or a couple of switches, it would necessitate our going down to Twenty-third Street to a place that carried all the Lionel accessories. It was a small, dark, narrow store, stuffed to the rafters.

The owner and Sam became friends. They discussed Sam's layout and whatever technical problems he was encountering as the complex grew and grew and had completely taken up all floor space in his room. One had to hop across bridges and trees to get to Sam's bed. I felt very fond of this man, who must have formed his own impression about the child who visited his store several times each week. He never asked; he simply greeted Sam joyfully when we walked in. I used to bring a book and sit and read while they had their consultation.

On the way home Sam was usually more cheerful, talking of the solution of his railroad problem or telling me that Dr. Zalinger had said that he had more tricks up his sleeve, not to despair, or—with a comical air—shaking his head, saying, "I wonder why Dr. Chevalier has this need to use bad language." I was delighted by the latter, finding that I enjoyed putting down shrinks now that my own analysis was over. I suppose that on some level, I understood both of these truths: that I was jealous of Sam's therapy and that Dr. Chevalier was trying to desensitize Sam.

On that same level, I think I also realized that Dr. Chevalier was seriously considering the possibility of surgery. And though, by agreement, the existence and nature of this surgery had not been discussed with Sam, through Sam the message was being piped to Mark and me. Except that we were not ready to receive it. During that year it was easier to act dumb, to cheer on Sam when he said something derogatory about Dr. Chevalier. In fact, I told that story about Dr. Chevalier's need to use bad language to all my friends! But it left an ache, a faint toothache in my brain; what I knew was not all that deeply buried.

MARCH 7, 1977

We are back with the gallows humor, laughing about "Martinez of Guggenheim." The story is not really funny; it's just that Rachel's I.V.s keep infiltrating—leaking—and have to be yanked out and then reestablished, and there is trouble in finding decent veins. The system here at Mt. Sinai is that a special team is responsible for dealing with everything concerning I.V.s. So a very nice woman comes and flinches when she sees that it's Rachel she has to stick again. And after two or three bad attempts, during which Rachel keeps reassuring her that it does not hurt at all and during which I go into the corridor, she wipes the sweat off her brow and says that she's going to send for Martinez of Guggenheim! Apparently he is her opposite number at the other pavilion; he comes to Klingenstein only at her invitation. Upon his arrival, we all make a great fuss. Today I told him that he is the king of the I.V. starters, but he says modestly—or diplomatically—that he learned everything he knows from his Klingenstein colleague.

Rachel is running a fever. Norma says it's nothing, not to worry, that no one thinks in terms of serious infection until the temperature goes over a hundred and one. By the time it did, Nanette was on. Oh, is she wearing better! I don't quite know what the affinity is, though of course Rachel and Nanette are close in age. And she is pretty and an aspiring actress. That's why she works the four-to-midnight shift, to be free mornings to go to auditions. Additionally, there is something straight and honest about her. I feel I can ask questions and get answers; she shares Rachel's passionate belief in the rights of patients to know the truth, to be treated with dignity. Mark put it well. He said the difference between Nanette and Norma is that Nanette allows the patient to be center stage.

I don't know how I could have left tonight except for Nanette. Not only because she is a good nurse, but because Rachel is less afraid when she is on. What is this lousy fever? What kind of infection? They are going to culture everything: urine, drainage, blood. Oh, God, please . . .

❦ ❦ ❦

The children were fighting constantly. A particularly nasty kind of quarreling. Sam would not let Rachel run the railroad; in fact, he would not let her into his room. True, she had been the cause of a crushed tunnel, and the milk cans had disappeared out of the dairy train. So they were at each other, and each, separately, at me. "Make him let me blow the whistle." "She's such a creep. Now she keeps complaining that she has cramps too." I explained to him that she was in need of some sympathy, and I explained to her that he was cross because he didn't feel well. Nothing helped. Once I came upon them in an actual melee, flying fists, kicking feet. I stood, appalled, then saw that Sam was not doing the hitting, was merely holding her off. But Rachel was slugging with all her might and screaming, "You're ugly, ugly. I hate you." In a sudden fury of my own, I yanked her away and slapped her face.

Telling Mark, I excused my excess by saying that I couldn't

bear how much she must have hurt Sam, whose skin was so taut and painful anyway. But later I knew that what had triggered me was her saying that he was ugly. The shock, the recognition, her lack of control, which threatened mine. Oh, how could she? I wept.

In the middle of the night she tugged me awake. I opened the covers and she crawled in, and I held her. Then she cried. "I didn't mean it," she sobbed. "I know you didn't. Hush, hush, don't wake Daddy." I stroked her face, her crisp curls. She whispered, "And it's true that I have cramps. Sometimes it hurts awfully. Sam won't believe me." I pressed her head against me; at last she dozed off.

Strange, this business with the looks. Here was Rachel at eight and a half and she could not bear Sam's disfigurement. And Mark, who would have sworn that he didn't give a damn how Sam looked temporarily, had abruptly given up his mania for taking movies. We made jokes about it, said thank goodness he's stopped following us around with that camera, and he replied that he was giving it up because he was tired of our lack of cooperation. But really, what was it? Had the sight of this Sam been such a terrible wound to his narcissism? And what about me? Why had I been handling those feelings with all that distance? Seeing Mark and Rachel react, but not myself. The feeling of walking into a store with Sam, and the iron discipline I had to apply not to explain, gush, say, "No, no, that's not the way he looks . . ."

So much for Dr. Paul Zalinger's ". . . parents will tolerate and even enthusiastically accept"! What Dr. Zalinger didn't understand was that the parents who agreed to try his wonder cure did so from a combination of ignorance and lack of choice. I wondered whether I would tell him so one day, then knew that probably I'd lack the courage. But possibly after a couple of drinks, feeling loose, saying, "Listen, Paul . . ."; the friendship was blooming. Mark had ignored my misgivings, my statement that it was not a good idea to get socially involved with our child's physician. And I hadn't been sufficiently convinced that it was all that "bad" to make my conviction stick. Or perhaps I was as eager for the friendship as Mark; I liked Nina, Paul's wife, a lot.

Rachel's complaints that she had cramps became a daily feature. It never occurred to me for a minute that they were anything except a bid for attention. And while I understood, sympathized, and wanted to help her also, I just couldn't stretch that far.

The latest on Sam was that he was not growing. Dr. Zalinger had taken x-rays to determine whether the epiphyses in his wrists were still open. Finding that they were, he explained that this was a good sign. As long as the epiphyses were unossified, there was a chance for Sam to catch up on his growing. But he was twelve now, and there was also the worry about his sexual development. When he was not incapacitated by the steroids, he was suffering the agonies of the disease. And it was a hell of a lot more disease than had been indicated by the phrase "smoldering symptoms," which kept lingering in my mind as something I had first read in Paul Zalinger's paper on Gustl's sofa. It had been two and a half years now since Sam had gotten sick and almost eighteen months that he was in Paul's care. Again and again a couple of other excerpts from that paper would come to mind: ". . . if the response to therapy is inadequate, surgical intervention should be considered . . . electively, if after a prolonged period, usually two years . . ." Time was running out, wasn't it?

It was sometime in April, because I remember that I had a riot of yellow-and-orange parrot tulips in my yard. I wrote a poem about God making my garden overspill, which rhymed with "child so ill" and ended with "are you crazy, are you crazy, God?" Yes, it was in April, and Sam was in the x-ray room, and Paul sat me down in his office and asked what I knew of the surgery. He was very gentle, none of his awful kidding; he said there was no urgency, but still. In Sam's case the advantage of elective surgery was that he was still young enough to catch up on all his growth and development and that psychological acceptance was better at his age. Anyhow, he said, Sam was special; Sam would handle it splendidly. But his colon was too far gone to save.

I was calm; after all, this was no surprise, and on top of it, it was only a dream; I would wake up out of this fall without hitting bottom. And now I could ask questions I had been suppressing. Amazed at my facility with the words, I asked him to explain how an ileostomy functions, what type of appliance the patient had to wear in which to collect body waste, how it would affect his life. I listened to the answers and knew that at last, I was taking them in. Oh, all the answers were reassuring—a completely normal life, a healthy life, growing tall, catching up—and I understood that now, soon, I would have to permit the clashing implosion and come to terms with the concept of "the same but different."

"Are you okay, Jean?"

"Yes, Paul."

And yes, I would pass the information on to Mark. Yes, of course he would want to speak to him in person. Yes, we would think about it. "Not too long," Dr. Zalinger warned.

That evening we had tickets to see *Fiddler on the Roof*. It was *the* show just then, and we were going with a crowd of friends. Somehow I survived the pretheater dinner conversation. Then we were seated, the house darkened, the thin music of the fiddle struck me, and, grasping Mark's hand, I burst into a torrent of tears. And wept throughout, wept and sometimes howled. "Listen to her!" one of our friends laughed; everyone thought I was really having a ball. Except, of course, Mark. Though there had been no time to tell him yet. During the intermission we stayed in our seats, he put his arm around my shoulder, and he didn't ask any questions. We would speak of it soon enough.

It was now certainly high time to tell Sam about the existence of the operation. Paul wanted to tell him during his next appointment. I felt the most incredible kind of dread and was unable to even imagine what kind of reaction Sam might have. "If you consider that it took me almost three years to come to a point where I can even acknowledge it . . ." For the first time I told Mark about my weird behavior after reading what it said in the Medical Encyclopaedia.

"In those green volumes?" he asked, pointing to the top shelf.

I nodded.

"Maybe," he said thoughtfully, "maybe it is the right decision to let Paul tell him. We'd load it with all our demons."

Still we argued with Paul, said that it was our place to tell Sam, but at last agreed when Dr. Chevalier also recommended the medical approach.

The day came, and it was our usual routine, both Sam and I in the waiting room, he with his history book, me staring at an article in *The New Yorker* which I had been trying for weeks to finish. Somehow I could never really take it in; this waiting was not conducive to concentration. After Sam had gone in, I found that it was even less possible on this occasion; my vision was blurred as well. I looked around, wishing to just be able to breathe past the lump in my throat. I envied the mailman who came, slapped down a bundle of letters, and left, and I felt an unpleasant empathy with the other people in the room—a woman my age who was whispering to an emaciated little girl, a teen-ager with the telltale pouchy cheeks, an old man with a tottery neck. Wanting to touch them, comfort them, at the same time that I wished not to be associated with them. What was Sam feeling now? Was Paul drawing him a diagram, showing him where on his abdomen there would be the outlet through which he would henceforth eliminate his body waste? The dread rose higher; it would crush me. . . .

"You can go in now, Mrs. Bergman." I walked down the corridor, my knees soft, the heat spreading up and down from the glowing ball in my middle. I tugged at my blouse to get it away from the clammy skin. Then heard Sam and Paul laughing. Paul was up, his hand reassuringly under my elbow. "Sit down, Jean." The pleasant room: a cool breeze from the air conditioner; blues— carpet and curtains; an antique medicine cabinet with many drawers with Latin names. Finally I looked at Sam, who appeared to be smiling. Impossible—the distortion of the steroid look; or me: yes, my perceptions were way off. . . . I tried to force myself to listen and actually heard much of it, Paul saying that Sam had, of course, reacted intelligently, understood, wanted to get it over with as soon as possible, be well—the deep voice resounding as if in a high-ceilinged chamber. Then Sam: "Mom?"

I met his eyes.

"Why didn't you tell me sooner?"

And later again, in the car going to the railroad place, but this time accusingly, "Why didn't you tell me, Mom?"

"I was scared," I replied.

"But I thought I would die."

Waves of shock in the car, my mouth parched, unable to say anything.

And then, incongruously, Sam laughed. "Man! I'm going to be all right." He rolled down his window, yelled into the New York din, "I'm going to make it!"

At Lionel, I bought him the Talking Station that afternoon. It said, "Last stop. All out!"

MARCH 10, 1977

I overheard an intern refer to Rachel as the "Pouch Princess." It was a shock, because it was funny. And, I suppose, apt. To see her O.O.B., as the chart says—*out of bed*—sailing toward me in the hall: tall; very straight, in her pretty robe; the long hair, still sun-bleached even now, down over her shoulders; one hand on the nurse's arm, the other pushing the I.V. pole; her output bags tied to her belt; the N.G. tube still in her nose—yes, like an exotic princess. And so damn dignified and beautiful. She smiles as she sees me coming; she is glad to see me, which doesn't mean that she is going to pamper me. Right off she points out the new bottle on the pole. Gentamycin, a different antibiotic: hopefully, she won't be allergic to it as she was to the Keflex. All the cultures have come back negative, but now there is talk of a wound infection. "Tomorrow it will be a week," she says, and suddenly there is discouragement and exhaustion; her voice gets even hoarser. "I have a hundred and two," she complains.

"Come on, Pumpkin," Nanette says. "Let's get you back to bed."

The return journey is less majestic.

MARCH 12, 1977

Rachel's strength is seriously sapped by the fever and the pain. She has a wound infection. The two rubber drainage tubes embedded on either side of the incision do not yield enough of the vicious fluid. Today they reopened a piece of the incision to permit more drainage. They poke and prod, hoping to break it up, make it flow out, bring down Rachel's fever. They also added Chloromycetin to the other antibiotic.

❦ ❦ ❦

Sam's Mother's Day contribution that year said, "Without you/I'd go cabloo/Be in a stew." He signed it, "Your loving kid, Sam." I needed the reassurance badly, because all our tempers were raw; even Mark was snapping at me. Because the mills had started grinding, and I had the feeling that I had made that first turn of the handle. Somehow, there was no way I could convince myself that I should not, in some way, have been able to prevent all this from happening. Mark felt the same way. We had endless intel-lectual conversations about it; we told each other that we were operating on the level of the stereotypical child who feels that *it* has caused the lightning to strike with its badness; we told each other that all things considered, we were pretty good parents, that we had no reason to give ourselves the added pain of this guilt.

But of course, the trouble was that there was no one else to blame. Obviously Dr. Zalinger's course of treatment had failed because Sam's disease process had been too far advanced already when we came to him. Well, and *if* we had come to him earlier? But we had not known of his existence until he published his paper. On the other hand, was the Genius from Yale responsible? How did we know that in the end, he was not correct in his way of looking at ulcerative colitis? After all, even Paul said that getting Sam to him sooner might not have made any difference—there *were* those three medical failures out of twenty! If Dr. Samuelson had been right, then why did we have to put Sam through the suffering of the secondary symptoms from the steroids? And were they really, truly, reversible? At that moment it was as difficult to imagine Sam normal as it had earlier been to picture him "mooned." Back and forth, again and again; Mark and I could find no peace.

Sam, however, was calm. His good feelings for Dr. Zalinger remained strong. It was just as he had known it would be; Dr. Zalinger would make him well; the surgery seemed to Sam a perfectly reasonable price to pay. Relieved as we were that Sam had this attitude, we also worried that he was too damn Pollyanna-ish about it, that there would have to be a terrible reaction at some point, that the almost eager way in which Sam seemed to anticipate putting up his dukes against that heavyweight agony was some form of masochism. Dr. Chevalier said nonsense to all of that. He repeated that Sam was doing the very best anyone could possibly do under the circumstances.

In the meantime, we had met the surgeon. A slight, sandy-haired guy with a pleasant manner and a warm smile, he was the antithesis of what we had pictured a surgeon to be. He was with Mark and me for two hours, sitting patiently, letting us ask every possible question, explaining, reassuring, sympathizing. He also made detailed drawings for us and referred to a chart of the human body during his explication.

What we learned was that Dr. Charles White was a pediatric surgeon, that he worked with two other surgeons, that they functioned as a team, which assured the patient of constant coverage. The surgery Sam required would be performed in two stages approximately a year apart. The reason for that was to cut down on the trauma by not resecting, or removing, the sigmoid (he pointed to the last section of the large intestine, just above the rectum on the chart) and the rectum (his pencil tapped it) at the same time as they would take out the colon. Here followed a long sweep of the pencil up the ascending portion of the colon on the right side of the body, across the transverse section just below the diaphragm going across the body, and down the descending colon on the left side. I shivered: that was an awfully big piece of intestine to resect.

Another reason, Dr. White continued, why it was expedient to do the surgery in two stages was that a chance existed that once the diseased colon was removed, the remaining rectal section would heal and could, at some later point, be reconnected. Again pointing: "Sew the healed sigmoid to the ileum. See?"

He showed us that the ileum was the winding mass of small intestines which lay higher up in the body. However, we were discouraged from counting on that because there existed only a very slim possibility for this outcome. In any case, at the time of the first surgical procedure, an ileostomy would be established on the right side of Sam's abdomen. This ileostomy would be the terminal inch of his ileum and would protrude from the wall of his belly about a quarter of an inch. Fecal matter would pass through it into an appliance that would be glued over it. This appliance would have to be emptied several times a day.

The listening was very difficult. There was the constant need to tune out, to watch the way the afternoon sun struck red in the stubble of Dr. White's hair, to wait for the second hand on the desk clock to jump ahead, to let the flow of Mark's and the doctor's voices stream past me and to fancy that they were of no concern to me. But somehow, I stayed with it. "The second operation," I said. "I mean, if he has to have it, is it as major as the first?" In the back of my mind, something I had read—that the operation is more dangerous for boys. I blurted, "Is there any danger—"

"Of impairing sexual functioning?" Dr. White finished for me.

We waited. Indeed, the surgical procedure was easier on females. A boy's pelvis is narrower, and the location of the prostate gland makes the resection of the rectum more difficult. "We cut very close to the nerve that is responsible for erection."

Mark had turned ashen. Dr. White added gently, "I have never had a problem." He emphasized the "never." Then there was silence. I began to gather my belongings, stuffed the cigarettes into my bag, found that my fingers wouldn't work. Idiotically, I tried to figure in my head how long I'd have to live with this terror. How old was a boy when he'd first have erections, emissions? Thirteen? Or earlier? How long until we could be sure?

Mark and I left Dr. White's office in a strange mood. We talked a lot about how impressed we were with the doctor, how capable he seemed, how nice he was, and that Paul's recommendation seemed absolutely justified. And of course, we knew that the operation was now imminent. Yet we still discussed it as if we had options: "If we decide," or "If it becomes necessary"—until suddenly a week later, the term "elective" was finally dropped from our vocabulary.

I had taken Sam to Paul's office for his regular appointment. It was May 19; Sam had been in very bad pain for a couple of days already. And when I was called into the office to join Sam and Paul, the doctor told me that Sam and he had just decided that the time had come.

I said, "I see." And then, "When?"

"Now." I felt hostile, considered telling him that shouting me down wouldn't get him anyplace, but, of course, didn't. Instead I argued that Sam needed pajamas, books . . . "His slippers," I said urgently.

Paul shook his head; then, still in a loud voice, said that he had decided, had already called the hospital, and though he couldn't get a bed on the floor he preferred at Children's, they'd transfer Sam there as soon as an opening became available. "I want him in today," he concluded.

And I understood that he considered it dangerous to wait any longer.

Admitting procedure meant waiting, sitting on long benches; everyone around us also sat, staring ahead, looking morose. Sam and I cracked jokes, hastily filled pockets of silence, finally played Who Am I? At last it was our turn, and Sam answered all the questions very efficiently. I sat by, then fought the sudden rise of hot tears as the plastic band bearing his name and newly assigned number was clasped around his wrist. He was an inmate. No, I told myself sternly, a patient. Cut the drama! I said, "Last time I was at Mount Sinai Hospital with you, Sam, *I* got the number; you were only 'Baby Bergman,' and the tag was around your ankle."

Sam refused the wheelchair, so we followed a page across the courtyard into an old building and up three floors in a rickety elevator. A very busy nurse in pink, looking like a nursery teacher, was adjusting a huge bandage around a scrawny neck. At the same time she warded off a skinny boy who was attempting to pull the little girl's six pigtails, and she kept murmuring, "Don't; don't, now, Frank," to a kid who was tugging at her skirt. We waited for attention. At last she looked at Sam's admitting papers. "Oh, yes; walk to Ten," she told us. "The last bed." As an afterthought: "Hi, Sam."

Ten had green walls and incredibly dirty windows, but the yellow curtains were fresh. There was a smell of greasy food: a woman was eating French fries out of a paper bag. "This is Joey," she said, pointing at her child, who had a grossly enlarged head. On another bed a slim girl sat holding a sleeping child's hand. His head was shaven; I turned away from the sight of the Mercurochromed cross over his temple. And next to Sam was Juan, who talked fast. "My mother comes later, maybe," he said. "I can manage alone."

"Sure," Sam answered. "My mom has to leave too."

I said yes, I would go, would buy pajamas, would be back.

"He don't need no pajamas," Juan advised. "They give them us." He pointed. At least, I thought, they are red; someone had veered off the institutional rail. Red, wrinkled, with drawstrings at the waist. "Well?" I asked, and waited. But Sam was looking at a comic Juan had offered him.

Outside, confused, I stood wondering what to do. Why had Sam sent me away? I called up Mark, who wore his busy voice. "I'll be there as soon as I *can*," he said and I, suddenly furious—excuse me for interrupting you, my Lord—answered, "No need! Just take care of your business as usual."

"Jean!" Through the tone of a man at his wit's end, a note of pleading.

"I'm sorry," I said, and meant it. There were excited, angry voices in the background. I could picture Mark behind his desk, see Ben and Phil and maybe others arguing around him, feel how he longed to make an island for himself and me. I said again that I was really sorry and that I'd go now and do some shopping and then be back with Sam. "Honestly, you needn't rush. It's a case of hurry up and wait."

I bought a pair of light blue pajamas with navy piping, the exact same kind Sam always wore. Then I got Silly Putty for all the kids in the room and *Classic Comics*. I hesitated before a big jigsaw puzzle of a gorgeous locomotive, but decided that it would take forever to put it together; it had too damn much of a feeling of permanence. As if I expected Sam to be there for a long time. Part of me argued that indeed he would be, but still I couldn't buy it. Instead I got a Hardy Boys book Sam hadn't read yet and funny noses and beards and gum. And back on the ward, found Sam, the fourth figure in wrinkled red, playing checkers with Frank, whose mama had since left and who was nodding the big head as if palsied. No, Sam didn't want the pajamas I'd bought; the ones he wore were fine. And, peeking into the paper bag at the other gifts, he decreed that I could only give out the gum. The sleeping child still had not awakened. I put his gum on his night table. His mother didn't say anything; it was as if she were also sleeping with open eyes.

Later, after Paul had come and drawn the curtains around Sam's bed to examine him, Sam motioned for me to leave them closed after Paul had left. I sat next to him as in a yellow tent. He whispered that Juan didn't have a telephone and thought that we must be rich because we did. He looked at me apologetically. "I didn't want to—" he began, and I answered quickly, "I understand. I shouldn't have brought all this junk." Then we just sat. Sam looked very tired; he was running a fever. But when Mark came they played chess on the little magnetic board Mark had brought. Later we couldn't believe the dinner tray: a slice of white bread in a waxed-paper envelope, a cone of deep-fried rice, a ball of mashed potatoes, a pile of corn kernels. And a gooey piece of cake. "Those starches!" I exclaimed. Sam hushed me. He couldn't eat anyhow.

The next morning on arriving I found Sam and his bed gone, and after my heart had stopped plunging, heard from the kids that he had been moved downstairs. I noticed that except for the boy who still slept they all wore the noses and beards. I said good-bye to them, took the elevator to the first floor, and stepped into a different world. A nurse in white smiled and led me to Sam's room, where he sat in bed, not only wearing the contested blue pajamas, but conversing with a tall, handsome boy who wore them in yellow. "This is Stevie Levy," Sam introduced. And in a stream: that Stevie had ulcerative colitis as well, that he was also twelve, that Dr. Zalinger was his doctor too, only Stevie hadn't been sick as long as Sam. In fact, he had had only this one violent exacerbation, but was bleeding so much that he had to be hospitalized.

"And Stevie says the food is neat down here. We get filet mignon."

"Only on Thursday," Stevie warned.

Weirdly, I was getting happier and happier as I listened to them. There seemed to be a great deal of relief in having Sam with someone who . . . well, what? Someone like himself? Someone of our "class"? I tried in my mind to say it in a comical way, in quotation marks, to make it ironic. So it would be as if I didn't mean it, as if it didn't count! Ugh—and didn't like myself.

Now a new pediatrician was added to the mix. A Dr. Bela Shelansky, who was said to have autocratic ways and a reputation as a brilliant diagnostician. We were prepared to withstand his advertised causticness, but found that he was very nice to us, though perhaps a little pompous. Probably Mark started us off on the right foot by first thanking him for taking Sam's case; deference was obviously in order. Then Mark and I exchanged raised eyebrows while Dr. Shelansky lit his pipe. Alas, in spite of the fun we were having with our little "manage-the-doctor" game, the pediatrician simply confirmed that the surgery was essential for Sam. In the meantime, he was to be built up for it. "How?" Mark asked, and got a mumble of technical terms. Dr. Shelansky was a believer in the medical mystique.

Walking back from his office, Mark said, "Built up! Like Hansel by the witch." I nodded; the image had occurred to me too. Hansel behind the fence—Sam with the crib sides of his hospital bed up. I said hastily, "The witch didn't give Hansel blood transfusions." "Is that what Sam will get?" "Well, I caught the word 'plasma.' That means blood, doesn't it?" "We'll ask Paul." We were meeting Paul and Nina for dinner. I had forgotten my opposition to the friendship; it was such a relief to have him be both friend and doctor.

Sam and Dr. Shelansky got on famously. True, there had been a moment when it could have gone either way—a morning when Sam suggested to the doctor that he ought to lower the Prednisone by five mg. To add to the tension of the acts of *lèse majesté*, there were witnesses—a nurse, an intern, and I. We all held our breaths. Then Dr. Shelansky nodded earnestly, pushed out his lower lip, nodded again, and said, "Very well, Dr. Bergman; I shall take your suggestion under consideration." After which he addressed Sam only as "Doctor" or "Colleague."

Sam's face was beginning to reemerge from the blubber. He had been at twenty milligrams when the last attack had started and when Paul had decided not to take him through another course of high dosage. So he looked more like a cute fat boy than a grotesque. But his legs were still very bad, the striations an angry red; they looked like very bad stretch marks. Another thing we found difficult to bear was that no date had been set yet for the surgery. We were told, "We are watching carefully" when we asked. What were they watching for? That his colon would not burst before he was "built up"? So it seemed. At last Paul explained that they were trying to boost his nutritional level, see that he had enough calcium, potassium, vitamins, etcetera. Yes, and blood too.

In the meantime, the boys' room was beginning to look like home: their own pillows and shams, a cactus someone had sent Sam in a Pluto pot, and Stevie's skinny avocado plant in a Maxwell House tin. Then there was Stevie's small fish tank—ignored by the authorities after initial shock—and the little T.V. we had bought Sam on which they were watching *The Fugitive* and the happenings at the Ponderosa.

They talked a lot about the space program: both fans of Grissom, Young, Schirra, and Stafford. Earlier, they had both watched the astronauts practice reentry in Gemini simulators and on March 23 had seen Grissom and Young land safely in the Atlantic in Gemini III. What drove them wild with delight, and was one of their favorite subjects for discussion, was that someone told them that this whole mission had been carried out to assess the effects of weightlessness on sea urchin eggs. Sam would copy Hubert Humphrey's send-off speech with additional material about the destiny of sea urchin eggs; he considered himself an expert on the Vice President because I had once sat next to him on a dais during an Israel Bond rally.

Then one morning when I walked in, I was shooed right out again. I stood trembling in front of the door, trying to recollect what I had seen: curtains drawn around Stevie's bed or Sam's? There had been so many people working over—yes, over Stevie. Where was Sam? And then I saw him down the hall in the entrance to the visitors' room. I hurried to him, put my arms around him; relief was making a buoyancy in my head.

Suddenly he was leading me to the settee, asking was I all right. Yes, yes; what happened? The boys had gone through the normal morning routine, had eaten breakfast, their beds had been made up, ". . . and you know, temps and medications and everything." But after the nurse had left, Stevie had told Sam that he had this

crazy pain in his shoulder. After a few jokes about ulcerative colitis that wandered around and hid in shoulders—next it would go
to Stevie's head, Sam had suggested—Sam had begun to realize that
his roommate was in serious pain. Over Stevie's protest, he had
called the nurse.

After that everything went berserk. The portable x-ray machine
and a million technicians and Dr. Zalinger and Dr. White and Dr.
Herbert and Dr. Shelansky and Dr. Gaon and all kinds of interns
. . . "I couldn't see what they were doing, but Stevie was choking
and moaning." Sam was crying now, sat next to me on the green
leatherette seat, dug his fists into his eyes. Then he said, "Until
someone remembered me and said to get me out of the room." He
jumped up, ran to the door, peered down the hallway. "What's
happening?" he called to a nurse who hurried past.

It was a while before someone told us that they'd taken Stevie
Levy to surgery. Not until Paul had come and explained did we
understand that the pain in Stevie's shoulder had been a dead-sure
indication of perforation. "Thank goodness that you called the
nurse," Paul said to Sam.

We spent the rest of the day waiting quietly, playing chess,
looking at T.V. Later we heard that Stevie was in the recovery
room. The next day he returned to the floor, but not to Sam's
room. He was in a single way down at the other end and Sam was
not allowed to go there.

"We don't want Sam to get scared," Paul explained to me, telling me that Stevie was very sick; it had been touch and go.

"Are you kidding?" I came back angrily. "Don't you think all
this secrecy is scaring him worse?"

Paul nodded, yes. And told Mark and me that perhaps, under
the circumstances, further waiting was counterproductive. So
Sam's surgery was set for June 3.

CHAPTER 4

JUNE 20, 1965

Reaction

Anxiety hurls me around
*   the empty atmosphere.*
Free fall through exhaustion,
*   ears black with roar,*
hurling past familiar holds,
without the wings of faith . . .
Unbound by gravity.

The world below is unreal, minute . . .
A child's toy, cracked calabash;
I have not even a parachute,
Can not land. I will smash.

MARCH 18, 1977

Looking back, it seems an indulgence, an enormous luxury, to have been able to relax into the kind of violent reaction expressed in the poem. Not this time. I am still together, bound by gravity. Things are not good enough to permit games. Every morning this week, when I get here around nine, I find Sam already sitting with Rachel. Apparently it isn't letting him be; he takes the subway from the Village, where he lives, then gets back to school in time for his first class at ten. He holds her hand and wills her to hang tough through these unbelievable days. When did it start to slip? My diary page for March 12 says that the Foley tube was removed at eleven A.M. and put back in the afternoon. That was last weekend. Two happy hours, symbolic of return to normal because the first of the mechanical supports had been removed. Hurrah, to pee on her own! I mean, we didn't say these things, we didn't make toasts; it was in the grins we exchanged. And in our anxiety when Rachel disappeared into her toilet. But she couldn't void, her abdomen started to distend, she was in pain. So they put the catheter back.

Okay, it was a little setback. Only on Monday she still had pain and was running a fever and her belly looked like a small hill. By Wednesday it was almost two weeks since the surgery, so, probably pushed by the timetable rather than reality, they removed the N.G. tube. Blessed relief, to be able to swallow without pain. On Thursday they took out the Foley again. There was an air of apprehension, though we celebrated with a day on liquids and a day on a soft diet. But today things blew.

Daniel and Ruth are here; they left the children with Ruth's mother. I tried to stop them from coming, told them that Rachel was not ready for visiting, but I guess they got too anxious, wanted to be with us, with her. And of course, I know that this business of my reluctance to tell them bad news is my hang-up. As if I were saying to Daniel, Don't be crazy, don't get mixed up in this, just be glad it didn't hit you too. The only one of my children not afflicted. Rachel reproached me, said that far from sparing him, I was shutting him out. So they came and walked right into the worst day: all the tubes are back in, plus a constant suction pump which is attached by a hose to the catheter in the pouch in order to keep the pouch empty.

The room is a jungle of wires and hoses and sounds, of machines going on and off, of lights flashing. N.P.O.—nothing *per os* (by mouth). All the cultures repeated, a gallium scan for abscesses, and another obstruction series, and Rachel in absolutely unreal pain which is hardly touched by twenty milligrams of morphine and a hundred milligrams of Demerol and something called Vistaril.

The big doctors are in and out all day as if it weren't a weekend. Dr. Gaon holds still for our questions outside the door, puts his hand on my arm, grins. "No, I'm not panicked like some people!" he says. I try to smile with him. Then he turns serious, looks terribly weary for a moment, adds, "Yes, I am concerned." What is causing the fever, the pain, what is going on inside—along the miles of sutures? Leaks, infections, obstructions, adhesions?

Other doctors contribute that they are not thinking of opening Rachel up again, not thinking of the O.R., not thinking of surgery. Lest we do! Apparently it is an obstruction in her intestines, but no one wants to say or knows from what. It could be scar tissue which is forming adhesions or the peel of the baked potato she ate yesterday. We kid her; I tell Daniel and Ruth that I have been assured that Rachel will go down in the annals of medicine as the only nut to eat baked-potato skin with her initial soft-diet meal. She tries to smile with us, but can't find a resting place—her back, her distended abdomen; she is holding on to Dan's hand; Ruth is perched at the foot of the bed; I leave the room. They are good with her, quiet and gentle and undemanding. I can see she's glad they are here. And Nanette just came in after reading the chart outside; still in her raincoat and holding her umbrella, she stood next to Rachel. The two girls looked at each other with tears in their eyes; then Nanette ducked down, put a small kiss on Rachel's arm, and said, "Stupid pumpkin."

Yes, better for me to be out of the room. I meet up with Mark, we walk the corridor up and down, everything is already familiar. The lady with anorexia nervosa, the amputee, the heart attack, the gall bladder, the other pouch patient at the end of the hall. She is only three days postop. "How is she?" I ask her nurse in passing. The nurse nods fine, fine. And I have a feeling of nostalgia for three days postop; Rachel was flying then.

🌷 🌷 🌷

Dan had offered to come home for Sam's surgery. We argued on the telephone; I said it was silly, he had just a couple of weeks to go before graduation, why should he miss out on the fun? "There's nothing you can *do* for Sam," I said. And added—more in an effort to produce the laugh that would ease us—"He's already taking his shrink into surgery; I don't think White would hold still for a brother as well!"

"He's what?"

"Honestly. Dr. Chevalier has asked Sam whether it would make him less afraid if he came along. Sort of a go-between, substitute parent among the doctors. Isn't that something?"

"I never heard of anything like that."

"Nor I. He's been fantastic. And somehow, it's making Daddy and me feel better too. He's promised to come out a couple of times to tell us how Sam's doing."

Dan asked, "And the surgeon said it was okay?"

I laughed. "It seems we have what is probably the only surgeon in captivity who's been in analysis himself. They say he used to haunt the hospital corridors at night, worrying about his patients. I mean, before he became 'well adjusted'! Anyhow, he understands. He's another one who's been terrific."

There was a pause. Then Dan said firmly, "I want to come home, though. I'll be with Rachel."

"All right." Suddenly I didn't want to protest anymore, didn't need to worry about Dan's absence from the pregraduation festivities, could let myself feel that I was glad that we would be all together; yes, it was right. It would be so much better for Rachel. She had lately taken to inviting friends for sleep-overs almost every night, but this buttress against loneliness did not suffice— late at night she'd come into our bed. She had cramps, a bad dream, she had to tell me something. "Psst, not now, in the morning," I would beg; I was ravenous for sleep. "No, no, you'll leave, you won't be here!" With terrible urgency. And I would listen. Yes, it would be wonderful for her to have Dan home.

He took her down to the hospital the day before the surgery and they stood in the courtyard—a very skinny tall young man and the curly-topped little girl—and waved up to Sam behind his dirty windowpane. We tried to open it for some shouted greetings, but it was stuck fast.

Then Sam got back into bed and became absorbed in the *New York Times* account of the next day's Gemini IV mission. For some time he had taken an inordinate interest in this flight. McDivitt and White were scheduled to take off at ten A.M. for their four-day, sixty-two-orbit adventure. Joshua Samson Bergman was also scheduled for takeoff at ten o'clock. And maybe, if the rocket stage sailed smoothly, Major Edward H. White II of the Air Force would float free on a tether in space. "Boy," Sam gloated, "he'll be propelling himself around with a space gun." The image of floating free as an euphemism for the anesthesia appealed to all of us. Mark, sitting on the bed with Sam, looked into the *Times* too. "But you'll be starting your descent at one P.M. already," he told

Sam. "When Ed White of the Air Force goes floating, Dr. Charley White of Mount Sinai has you pegged for a two-o'clock reentry." They laughed.

And then it was the day. After the poem was started, it was only seven o'clock, and Mark was finally in an uneasy sleep. I stared at the sunny seascape by Kitty Brandfield that hung across from our bed, but it didn't provide the customary lift. There simply is no help, I told myself firmly. Not in a beautiful painting, not in conjuring up a scene of all of us at the beach when this will be over. Nothing will help right now; the feeling has to be endured.

Thinking that, I remembered back to the separation from the analyst and how, after the termination date had been set, I would arrive each morning, plop down on the couch, and begin to weep. It had been quite marvelous. At last, at forty, I had given in, felt pain, permitted myself grief. But I had presumed that I had won a lasting victory, that from then on and forevermore I would be accepting of my feelings. Which had not turned out to be true; over and over, especially in these last months, I had kept coming up against denial. If I made a joke, if my mouth was stretched into a smile and my eyes sparkled, surely that meant that all was well. Yes? No? Which was why, that morning, I needed to tell myself to stop the waste motion, to stand still, to endure.

I moved close to Mark, put my arms around him gently. "It's time to go," I whispered. And felt consciousness hit him like a bullet, felt his body recoil, felt his pain with absolute empathy. But said again, "Come on, we have to go." Yet we lay still a little longer, savoring the comfort of touch.

At the hospital, Sam greeted us absentmindedly—he was absorbed by the T.V.; declared angrily that they were having trouble with the damn overspeed regulator of the erector. There were a lot of people in and out of the room—things were being done to Sam, and we kept being asked to step outside—but Sam ignored all that; he had focused his anxiety on Cape Kennedy. "It's an electric failure," he told us the next time we came in.

"What the hell is an overspeed regulator?" I asked angrily. While we were in front of the door, we had heard Sam cry out in pain; they were inserting the catheter.

"It's a thing that's supposed to keep the erector from dropping too fast. But right now it's keeping it from lowering at all."

A nurse stood by with a hypodermic. "Just one more, Sam," she apologized. "It's Vitamin K."

"That's to keep you from bleeding excessively," I said, happy to recognize this good vitamin from my sole hospital experience of childbirth.

Sam turned his hip to the nurse, but kept on explaining that the erector was a hundred-thirty-ton tower hinged to the launch pad, that it had to push the Titan II missile to the upright position.

On the screen McDivitt and White stalked about, grotesque pandas. In Sam's room a green-clad attendant arrived pushing a long stretcher and said to Sam, "Well, pal, wanna take a ride?" However, the nurse waved him out again, explained that the patient was not ready. To me, indignantly, "His tube isn't in yet." We stood and waited. Until a young doctor arrived whom Sam seemed to know and who promptly sent us packing once more. As we were leaving, I heard Sam say, "But listen, Dr. Gaon, take it easy, take it slow; I can't take off before they do." Then the door closed. "Who's he?" Mark asked, and a passing intern told us that it was Gaon, the chief surgical resident; he'd finish prepping Sam.

Suddenly Sam was on a stretcher under a green sheet. There was a tube in his nose and an I.V. in his arm, and he was very, very sleepy; he smiled at us. We walked next to him to the elevator and waited there till it came, and Mark kept stroking Sam's hand and saying, "Don't worry, don't worry." Sam murmured back, "Watch 'em." I realized that he meant the astronauts only after he was gone. Then I was sorry that I hadn't promised him that we would. So Mark and I went back to the room obediently. It was being cleaned, transformed. All the syringes, the plastic wrappings, the cotton, the gauze, the rubber tubing, and the blood-soaked swabs were gone; it was a sterile, impersonal room with an empty bed.

I wrote the second part of the poem and watched T.V. while Mark stared at the *Times*. Once he told me that Arab guerrillas had raided Israel twice the previous night. At eleven fifteen McDivitt and White finally got off, and at twelve Dr. Chevalier, all in green, came down to say that the operation was going well, that the colon was out—"and high time, too." Then, answering the quick panic that must have jumped into my eyes, he added, "No, no, White is sure it's clean. It's just all burned out!" He also said that Sam was in absolutely first-class shape.

After he left, Mark and I came together, stood holding each other. Neither of us had discussed with the other how much the fear that malignancy would be found in Sam's colon had been a part of us. And even now, "White is sure it's clean" wasn't all that reassuring. Yet we knew that it would be days until the pathology report would be back with a final answer.

So we simply held on to each other; there was nothing to be said. And then went back to watching the T.V. screen. Because of their delayed takeoff, Ed White had not floated in space at one o'clock as planned; in fact, we missed seeing him do it while talking to Dr. Chevalier. But I heard that it had been audible from earth when he exclaimed, "I'm doing great; this is fun!" in sufficient time to report it to Sam when we met once again at the door of the elevator. He looked beautiful, pink-cheeked, more normal than he had in months; it was all over.

The nurse was young and quick. Every time I came into the room during the night, she was doing something for Sam—adjusting the I.V.s, taking his blood pressure, wiping his face, talking to him in a low voice. I would go back to my bed on the green leatherette love seat in the visitors' room reassured.

Sam made a triumph of each day's climb back up. He was in a race with himself; when Dr. White predicted that the ileostomy would start to function on Thursday, Sam said no, on Wednesday. The reason it would take a few days before the ileostomy could be expected to work was that the peristalsis—the natural successive waves of involuntary contractions passing along the walls of the intestines—which forced matter through had been paralyzed by the trauma of the surgery and was being kept sluggish by the morphine and other painkilling drugs that had to be administered during the first days. But indeed, Sam made it a day ahead of schedule, and he and Paul laughed gleefully as if they'd known all along that Sam could do special tricks.

Mark and I were swept along by this stampede of pleasure. The sight of the first trickle of waste flowing through the ileostomy into the plastic, see-through bag that was glued over the stoma on to Sam's belly was one of pure joy and gratitude: it worked. Yes, a person could live without a colon. More dreaded, the moment of first seeing Sam's cut-up belly, also turned into a kind of victory. I'd been willing to postpone it; had volunteered to leave the room when the surgeons came to change the dressing; had said, eagerly, "I'll step outside." But Sam had commanded imperiously, "No, stay!" And watched me like a hawk lest I look away, lest I flinch.

After the first shock it was okay, quite neat. "Nice sewing," I could say sincerely, and join the banter between the doctors and Sam. And then felt elation because Sam had made me brave. He also made everyone else toe the line, suggested reduction in the painkillers as he felt better, watched over the change of dressing the scar. One day he stopped Dr. White from using the wrong tape. "That stuff hurts!"—pointing to the roll in Dr. White's hand. "You're right; I'm sorry," Charley White acknowledged, and he sent for the ouchless adhesive.

Sometimes I worried, afraid that some nurse or young doctor would misunderstand, would find Sam's relentlessness obnoxious, would not understand Sam's determination to facilitate his recovery to the utmost. But I needn't have worried: the staff on that floor was quite extraordinarily involved; everyone pulled with Sam.

Miss Baker was a small blonde who came on evenings. She was the one to administer several of the shots that fell due at the low point of the day. One evening she was met by a stream of water as she approached Sam's bed with the medication in her hand. Aghast, I yelled, "Sam!" He had filled a used hypodermic with water from his pitcher—he had a collection of them, needles broken off, and he was going to be the kid with the most water guns in the neighborhood! Apparently something had snapped in Sam at that hour and he had decided that he had to shoot back.

Miss Baker stopped short, wiped her uniform, then said evenly that she'd clobber Sam if he did that again. Sam said, "Sorry." Then, silently, she gave him his injection. But before leaving, she stopped at the half-finished jigsaw puzzle on the table and, searching for a moment, picked a piece and fitted it into place. "There!" she exclaimed, and grinned at Sam. He shouted, "You're terrific!" which might have referred to her good eye. The locomotive puzzle I had finally bought was a bitch to put together.

Stevie, down the hall, was still very sick. He was fighting infection caused by his perforated colon. No one was actually speaking of peritonitis, but apparently that was what they were dealing with. It surprised me that Sam didn't insist on being allowed to visit his pal—the daily walks he was now taking along the corridor could have been stretched to Stevie's door. But one day he remarked to me that he kept realizing how lucky he had been to have the surgery electively rather than in an emergency situation, and I realized that the jungle tom-toms had reached him about his former roommate's condition. He apparently felt that parading his own superior progress would increase Stevie's burden. Everything was going by the book for him—the ileostomy functioning, the scar healing, being able to urinate without the aid of a catheter—all the taken-for-granted functions were returning to normal. Sam was aware and grateful; he was saying thank-you prayers.

There were no secrets on the floor. We knew everything about everyone. We knew that Liza had become almost vegetablelike as a result of a weird accident in the O.R. She had been anesthetized for a routine test, and something had gone wrong. When we joined the first-floor community, Liza could not walk or speak or see. In the next six weeks, the time of our stay, we witnessed a near-miracle. She had the most amazing nurse, who worked with her incessantly. A worn, middle-aged woman, aggressively unattractive, whose harsh "Yes, you can, Liza. Yes, you can do it!" rang along the corridor for hours every day. She first dragged, later walked eight-year-old Liza up and down, up and down, endlessly. My early squeamishness at watching the terrible struggle left me, and it became a daily necessity to know how Liza was. One morning as I arrived I met the nurse and she told me that Liza could see and I broke into a torrent of tears. Running to tell Sam, I found that he knew already. We hugged happily. I said, "That nurse! God, she was radiant. Who would think that she could look almost pretty?" Sam, surprised, answered, "What do you mean? She's always pretty."

We also knew that Rico had leukemia. A most beautiful little boy who flew along the hallway in his Superman cape and whose lovely young mother spent hours each day teaching him how to read. "Pay attention, Rico," she would say sternly. "What kind of a man will you be if you don't know how to read?"

The boy in the wheelchair also had leukemia. White-faced, with a puffy body, the steroid look. He sat quietly and watched the other children play. His mother was as shy, as colorless as he. That was a strange thing—there we were, watching each other's dramas, involved with each other's children, and I, for one, wildly admiring the kind of heroism exhibited by some of those parents, but we did not really come close to each other. Just the smiles and nods and How is Sam today? To which one replied with either a "fine" or a little shake of the head. One did not pour one's heart out to the other, one did not place additional burdens; everyone had as much as he or she could bear.

At night, at home, there was Rachel. After Dan left, she had gone into a tailspin, not wanting to go to school, crying, fighting. All I could do was arrange for a close friend of mine whom she loved to spend time with her. Dan's graduation was on the thirteenth. Mark went up to Brandeis; I stayed with Sam. No doubt Dan must have been relieved to get back into his own life after the stint with Rachel; she had given him a horrible time, clinging fiercely, angrily demanding. Innocently, he had tried to oblige, only increasing the conflict; there was no satisfying this kind of need.

It must have been tough for him to handle his anxiety about Sam, his desire to help Rachel which had turned sour, and the flock of little girls she had inflicted on him all at the same time. Rachel had continued to bring home sleep-over and eat-with-us guests, telling Dan in a manner of no great subtlety that his efforts to satisfy her were insufficient. I had observed all that and promised myself that I would attend to it when this was over; Rachel will be all right until then, I thought, and I did not worry about Dan.

If I had thought about it, I might have said that I fancied myself an athlete in prime condition at that time. Part of this conditioning was the ability to concentrate. I was trying to eliminate anything that broke my concentration, I was rationing my strength, and I was ruthless in ridding myself of the social niceties that attend sickness. So I had asked Mark to stand between our mothers and me. Their anxieties were certainly legitimate, but I could not handle them at that moment. I had just enough strength for the things I considered essential—such as always having a funny story in the morning and staying calm and being willing to work on the puzzle with Sam.

Aside from the grandmothers, the visitor question was fairly simple. We just informed everyone that Sam was not to have company; then we made exceptions. Actually, Sam wanted to see our close friends, or maybe he wanted to be seen by them; what fun to be a hero without an audience? One couple, going to a costume party clad in Chinese outfits of some magnificence, sneaked in late one night via the basement labyrinth of corridors. Sam enjoyed that, not least of all because hospital rules were being broken. Another friend of mine popped in every afternoon after her analytic session; she would stay for ten minutes (forty-five, plus ten, plus five minutes to get to the meter), and Sam incorporated these mini visits into his routine. The only problem was the rabbi. Sam loved him and he loved Sam, which made it incredibly emotional —the very thing I could not handle. "I can barely manage myself;

how the hell am I to deal with the rabbi's tears?" I yelled at Mark. Mark didn't know.

Of course, after four, five weeks of this, we were pretty tired. Each morning the effort of getting out of bed was greater. And yet I knew that I would have to pace myself, that I had to keep a reserve for the end sprint, that the real demands on my strength and wisdom would be made when Sam came home. Also, the first euphoria had worn off. Yes, Sam had come through the surgery well; yes, the pathology report, which had arrived at last, bore out that there was no malignancy; and yes, Sam was recovering in a sensational way; but now we would have to learn to cope on a daily basis. With the end of private-duty nurses, Sam was exposed to the natural coming and going of the floor nurses. While "Children's One" rated excellent people, Sam was now seeing new faces, personalities not as involved as the first team had been.

One of the main things that concerned us was learning to attach the appliance over the ileostomy. The hospital used disposable, see-through plastic bags which had a cardboard disk on top. This disk had an opening that fitted over the ileostomy and was backed by adhesive which made it adhere to the body. The "disposables" were changed daily, and we were advised to use them for a while after going home before switching to a heavier appliance which would then have to be changed only every week or so. The heavier, or "permanent," appliances were made of rubber, had the shape of a pear, and were the size of a child's football. Their disks were hard rubber, and the adhesive used on them came in a tube and had to be applied to both the disk and the skin.

Sam and I, trying to learn the technique of the procedure, watched the nurses carefully. Both of us were anxious about the day when we'd have to manage alone. One of the nurses was very helpful when she explained that once Sam was strong enough to stand securely in the bathroom, he could do it himself much more easily than it could be done by another person while he was lying down. This promise of independence was extremely reassuring. Just the same, at that moment the whole business appeared to be a rather high mountain to climb.

One morning a completely strange nurse appeared and proceeded to shoo me from the room. In the past, there had ensued an unspoken struggle between Sam and me at such moments—I always quite willing to be dispatched, Sam determined to have me stay. Now I understood more and more that Sam was using Mark and me to test reactions to his new physical being, and I realized that it was terribly important that I show no desire to escape.

Accordingly, I told the nurse that I would prefer to stay and watch her change the appliance. She faced me, arms akimbo, declaring that mothers were a nuisance, upset the children, and made the nurse nervous. I, with heart beating rapidly, not sure whether from anger or from fear, said that nevertheless I would remain since, when Sam was home, it would be his mother he would look to for help until he could do it himself. After which the "fierce one," as we came to call her, ignored me, and not saying another word, expertly changed the appliance. Leaving me feeling wrung out.

Strangely, in the remaining weeks at the hospital, we began to like each other, exchanging first tentative smiles, finally a few jokes. She was on duty when Sam left, and while I took no note of the emotion at that moment, we later reconstructed that she had given Sam a brisk hug and shaken hands with me. "Who would have thought—" I began, and Sam, entertaining Mark, broke up: "Oh, oh you should have seen Mommy the first time 'the fierce one' let her have it!"

A poem I wrote before Sam came home is one of the survivors. Again, not for excellence of form, but because of the validity of what it said—that it was time to leave the hospital nest, time for back to normal, time to go home. And in the almost unconscious way in which I let those poems spill out, said; "never mind that you are altered . . . sensitivities, rife with new status, it's time to go home," I was relieved of anxiety and did not really have to think ahead to Sam's giving up his place at Children's, where he was a winner, and certainly not to the day when Sam, back at school, would reenter the locker room. Only much later did it occur to me that writing a wise poem did not connote wisdom; that these unexplored pieces were spillage that permitted me to deny quite effectively. I wrote it, ergo, I understand! Not so.

The weather was glorious, hot and dry, the first weekend Sam was at home. We sat in the garden under the oaks. I remember swimming in relief. For certainly we had survived the hardest period of our lives. It seemed just then that nothing bad would ever happen again, and any thought of a second operation was effectively erased; I would always feel this absolute beatific splendor. When Rachel came running up the hill, puffing from the exertion, her round face glowing and pink, I hugged her to my side. It was so lovely to be home with her, not to have to run and run and run, not to be split asunder. "Where have you been, love?" I asked.

"Kenny has the chicken pox."

"Stay away from him."

"Okay." A little pause, then, "Mommy? I just played with him."

"You what?" A terrible rage was rising in me. I grabbed Rachel, must have looked fearsome; she cowered while, at the same time, trying to pull away. "That woman let you in?" A scream.

"I told Mrs. Foster that I've had them."

"But you didn't." I was still shrieking; the fury was directed at the nice Gert Foster two houses down: How could she do this to me? How could she let Rachel into her house when Kenny had the chicken pox? Why was she after me? Oh please, please, what would I do . . .

Mark was out of his chair. He pried my fingers off Rachel's arm, he pulled her close to his side, he spoke soothingly to her, to me. But I didn't hear what he said. I sat down in the grass and howled. Dear God, how I cried.

MARCH 21, 1977

Today they have removed the Foley catheter again, but Rachel is depressed. The last few days were bad. Acute pain, N.P.O., repeated obstruction series, blood drawn for calcium tests—blood drawn, in fact, for every damn test in the book. And there was the night which I did not witness, the night about which Rachel tells me in dribs and dribbles. Not because she didn't want to tell me before, but because she couldn't. And because, much of the time, she is either in too much pain or too drugged to talk. Her eyes are huge in her face; she tries to smile. "Thank God Nanette was on that night," she says.

Nanette had gotten Dr. Gaon to come back to the hospital at some ungodly hour, and the internists had been there as well. A lot of doctors were milling around the x-ray room, but when the x-ray table was swung into the vertical position, Rachel had passed out. She doesn't remember what happened next. She does, however, recall the way the stretcher rushed down the corridors, the whir of the elevator, the unreality of being trapped in her body. Her alien body, more hated than ever before. "And I have hated it some!" she says, and inspects the part of the incision that is still open, is still being poked and prodded, while the rest of the scar is already a thin red line. "Look," she complains, "this will never heal together as nicely as the other part. They can't resuture it." I make soothing noises, trying not to show my terrible empathy. Though today she is better, less distended, it seems as if she has run out of will. And it is pouring outside.

In the morning I tried to ignore Rachel's mood and did my normal stint of gardening; the plants are thriving by the tall hospital windows, which have yielded an increased light level after I again tackled them with Windex. Then a general cleanup. Norma is getting to be a trial—her scattered things, her private telephone calls, her soap operas. We have tried lightly, jokingly, asking whether she couldn't adjust to *our* soap operas, but her insensitivity is hintproof. Especially when Rachel is feeling ill, the noise and confusion bother her. So it's easier for me to simply restore calm, pick up the mess, and encourage Norma to take another coffee break. But this morning, far from creating relief, I am bothering Rachel as well. She tells me to stop fussing, sit down; no, she doesn't want her back rubbed. Then, with tears in her eyes, "Yes I do. God, it hurts. Mom, do you mind?"

"Of course not," I say, so glad that there is something I can *do*, and go at it slowly, rubbing and patting and kneading, varying the movement of my fingers to defeat their fatigue. I wish I had more strength in them. The room is quiet. Soon the Ben-Gay smell permeates it; the windows stream. When I can't go on, I sit down. Rachel's eyes are closed, but she is not sleeping.

After a while she goes to the bathroom, pushing her I.V. pole with her. Announcing success, she tries to grin when she comes out again. But my quick flare of relief that this is working is muffled in her listlessness. Even when she gets a telephone call from one of her friends she is not cheered. I begin to wish that Dr. Freund would come soon. It's childish of me, I know: a psychiatrist has no magic to dispense; supportive therapy is just what the name implies; the actual lifting of the burden Rachel has to do herself. Yet I am glad that she decided to have this support during the weeks of making the decision to go ahead with the surgery. To me, acquainted only with the stylized ritual of psychoanalysis and the silent analyst, this warm young shrink seems very comforting. Yet from the little Rachel discloses, he's got her zeroed in on herself quite traditionally.

Endless day. The surgeons come and go, then the internists. Rachel reports that the pain is less, then complains about the N.G. tube: it's choking her; her throat is raw.

"Tomorrow maybe," Dr. Gaon holds out. Then asks, "Hey, what's the matter?" He's referring to the absence of her usual persona.

"Just feeling shitty," she admits, and taps herself on the forehead.

Later Dr. Freund helps her after all. Quite spectacularly, in fact. He crossed the several blocks between his office and the hospital in a torrential downpour, arrives absolutely drenched, his pants sticking to his legs, his hair in his eyes, the proverbial drowned rat. And Rachel takes one look at him and breaks into peels of laughter.

God bless spite.

❧ ❧ ❧

Rachel's case of chicken pox was also spectacular. What's more, she had it at our next-door neighbors' down the hill, whose children were away at camp. Paul and Dr. White had advised us not to expose Sam. So Rachel moved in with Naomi and Arthur and came down with it right on schedule and had a virulent case. I would look back to that moment under the trees when I had thought that I was done running and being split asunder. Now I really ran. Up and down the hill: time for Rachel's temp; back to irrigate Sam, change dressings, appliance; down to Rachel to sponge her; up for Sam's lunch; Rachel's aspirin; Sam's need to talk; Rachel's tears. Everyone was wonderful: Naomi and Arthur and their housekeeper and our Caroline. But still, there was this Mommy thing. At night, at last in bed, Mark would hold me carefully, since I was aching from tiredness, and we'd get slap-happy with the awfulness of it. "And otherwise how did you like the play, Mrs. Lincoln?" Mark asked. We would laugh and then I'd preach, "You know this isn't a tragedy, just a nuisance."

Oh, but it was the straw.

Finally we did get to the beach. We were back at the house in Hampton Bays. Happiness. Sam was ready to swallow the world whole. He was changing his appliance by himself; he answered questions about how he was feeling with an impatient shrug; in fact, I had to trust my observations rather than his reports. He was almost off the steroids now—it had taken this long to accomplish the gradual reduction that was designed to avoid his going into adrenal shock—and he was still a little heavy and mooned. But raring to go, to play tennis, to swim. Only I observed how quickly he would tire. I called the doctor about it, described how it looked to me as if Sam kept running out of steam a lot.

"Yes," Paul acknowledged. "Yes, I was just going to call you. His last blood tests show a slight case of hepatitis. You know, hepatitis is often an aftermath to blood transfusions . . ." He hesitated, then asked, "Do you know anything about hepatitis?" Hell, yes, I thought; a friend of mine had died of it. But Paul was approaching it so carefully, was trying hard not to scare me. "Honestly," he said, "Sam's case is probably already over now." More reassuring than his words was that he did not curtail Sam's activities, that he insisted it was more important for Sam to have some fun now. So the only obeisance we made to the hepatitis was an afternoon nap. And Sam did get stronger day after day.

Then, on a rather nasty weekend at the end of August, the Zalinger family came to visit. Rachel chased around with their two girls; Sam and Paul decided that they had to go swimming.

"But it's too cold," I protested, and was ignored.

At the club pool, they stood next to each other, the knobby man with the wild gray hair flying in the wind, the round-faced boy. Both had goose bumps, but by then Nina and Mark and I had caught on to the weight of the moment. Here was the redemption of a solemn promise. True, it had never been verbalized, but Paul's commitment to it had been as serious as Sam's trust. Paul would see Sam well. And here they were, at the pool together. Sam, forbidden to dive, glanced up at Paul, then dived into the water. Paul followed. The observers at poolside sniffled.

When we discussed it later, it was agreed that the chances Sam felt he had to take were absolutely essential to him. "Anyhow," Paul said, "if you noticed, he took a deep dive—not a chance of a belly-flopper; Sam is no fool."

In September he was back in school, seventh grade. At first he had to work pretty hard to catch up, but after a while his grades settled into their normal groove. Sam was an A-minus–B-plus man. I had a theory that people achieve at a level on which they are psychologically comfortable. To Sam it was important not to be thought of as a grind—especially now, when he fancied himself a jock, certainly a future jock. *Just let me get really well, then watch me go!* In any case, I had informed the school that Sam, while allowed to take gym, was not to be involved in contact sports. Later I found out that the coach had taken him aside on the first day and offered the use of his office if Sam would prefer not to change with the other boys. Sam had refused.

Exactly what happened that day in the locker room he never told us, but certain things leaked through—a boy said his scar was gross; another laughed. Sam, when asked about it, answered all questions with a wild tale of his exploits in the Foreign Legion. It was clear that he felt no more comfortable with taking his peers into his confidence after the operation than before. Once, when I spoke to him about trusting people, he gave me a strange look, as if to say, *Are you kidding? Don't you know how rough it is out there?*

Mark and I worried about it. Was it Sam's nature to be solitary, or had he suffered some abysmal experience that had convinced him that he could not risk opening himself up to people? Regardless, he had this dictum: only family was to be trusted. I longed to hear Dr. Chevalier's commonsense comment on all this, but Sam had discontinued the sessions with him. At his first appointment following the summer vacation, he had simply informed me that Dr. Chevalier and he had decided that he did not need any more therapy.

It was a busy fall. Mark was in his second term as president of the synagogue. Sam was studying for his Bar Mitzvah in March; Hebrew school was taking big bites out of his time. Rachel juggled a social life that was unbelievable with Hebrew, piano, painting, and tennis lessons. All of which kept me chauffeuring constantly in addition to my community commitments. Deliberately, we were involved, hectic, normal. Because there was no more doubt that the second stage of the surgery would have to be performed. "No rush, of course," Paul had reassured us. But he had also said that the continuing low-grade disease in the remaining intestinal section was preventing Sam from getting his growing spurt and was keeping him from feeling really well. "Which is why we may as well get it over with in the spring," he concluded. And lit his cigar.

"I won't even think of it until after Sam's Bar Mitvah," Mark countered sharply. He too lit up. Minutes ago they had been talking about trying these Coronas. I watched and thought of what had been said; I nodded—oh, yes, literally, Mark and I refused to think about it. Not yet. And weren't we entitled to this respite, to some pleasure? And wasn't Sam?

"What shall we do Thanksgiving?" Mark asked one night.

The kids shouted, "Williamsburg!" For years we had tried to take this outing; each time it had been prevented by sickness. Now was the time. "Don't fall out of any trees," Mark warned all of us.

So we visited the historic sites, and Sam wore a tricornered hat and carried a musket, and Rachel had a bonnet and stuffed Sam's rolled-up jeans under her robe to give herself a crinoline effect. Dan joined us and announced that he was going to get married, and all of us gorged on spoon bread: the American family having Thanksgiving dinner at the hearth of an old inn. Good things were ahead.

Good things like Nassau for Christmas and New Year's. And then in January, Paul and Nina went down to some islands. In the past, while Sam had been so ill, Paul had always left me his itinerary. He offered it again, and I remember taking it with some shame; I should let go of these crutches, I told myself. On top of which Mark had to be in Europe on a business trip at the same moment. Anxiety time for me. "It's the mass exit of the rats," I complained. But was told that no ship was sinking, and of course, they were right.

Except, it turned out, they were wrong. On a Wednesday morning, Rachel complained of cramps. I followed my usual routine: took her temperature; prepared to tell her again, as I had done regularly once or twice a week during the last months, that she had no fever and could go to school and that the cramps would get better as soon as she was busy. But that morning she did have a little temperature elevation, and I saw that she was pale. Oh dear, which? Measles, mumps? A quick panic inside—would Sam catch it? Then, laughing at myself: probably a little cold. Or indeed, an upset stomach.

Rachel was watching me. "Yes, you can stay home," I said. I half expected that she would protest now that she had won my attention, but she lay back in bed, obviously relieved. She was holding her belly. "You really do feel bad?" I asked. "I told you!" I bent down, laid my face next to hers, nuzzled her, but suddenly she was pushing me aside, rushing up, out of bed and into the bathroom. Seconds later I heard the sounds of explosive expulsion. Oh, dear, she did have an upset stomach. And then her cry, "Mommy, I have blood!"

"Stop it!" I yelled. Anger twisted my stomach; this was getting ridiculous. All very well to be psychologically understanding, to know that she needed to copy Sam, that she was fighting for her moment in the sun, the little idiot! But what about us? We couldn't be expected to be this goddamn understanding forever. The very thought of blood in a stool was making me ill, and I realized that the thing twisting my stomach was not anger, but fear. Sure, that's what she intended—to scare me good. I heard her crying in the bathroom and called harshly, "Just stop that, Rachel."

"Mommy!" Really pitifully. "Please come in."

I marched with heavy step, prepared to be severe. This had to stop. But in the door was assailed by a smell I knew—oh, God, the horrid, sweet smell I knew so well. I felt myself now going cold after the heat of anger, felt my knees wobble, looked past her bottom into the toilet bowl and saw the expected sight. Suddenly I was calm, pushed the hair off her damp forehead, said, "It's nothing; don't worry," and handed her the toilet paper. She was watching my face. She asked, "Do I have it?"

"Do you have what?" And with a little laugh, "Don't be silly." Then, "Come on, let's get you back to bed. You have a virus."

When she was back in bed, I returned to the bathroom. The smell was fainter, but unmistakable. I opened the window, caught sight of my face in the bathroom mirror; oh, how I hated myself with that drawn look. I walked quickly to the phone to call Dr. Freeman, only to be reminded by the nurse that it was Wednesday, his day off. No, I didn't want to talk to anyone else. Could she leave word for him to give me a ring if he should call in; it was kind of urgent. The nurse couldn't promise. After that I stood, looked around, found it hard to know what to do next. An incoming telephone call took my mind back to the meeting I would have to attend that afternoon; I was cochairing a charity luncheon. I talked about it with my caller, and then, after hanging up, continued to think about it. I'd have to get hold of the caterer and see the florist. And the reservations were coming in too slowly; we'd have to form a follow-up telephone squad. And the seating. I hated that job; maybe Naomi would do it.

"Mommy?"

"I'm coming, Rachel."

"Did you call Dr. Freeman?"

"It's Wednesday; he isn't in."

"What are we going to do?"

"Do? Nothing, love. I'm going to make you a nice cup of tea and get you the heating pad, and then you can watch T.V. Tomorrow you'll be fine." Should I call Paul? Nonsense. What could he do? I must not panic.

"I hurt."

I sat down on her bed, pulled her close, held her. I whispered, "I know, I know." She felt heavy against me; I also smelled the familiar odor of illness and fear on her skin. Anxiety rose in me like a tide, and I laid her back against her pillow and soothed, "It will stop. Honestly!"

When I left the house, I asked our housekeeper, Caroline, to spend some time with Rachel. She had had several more bouts of diarrhea. I was taking note of the well-known rush of feet, the slam of the bathroom door; but I was not connecting these aural impressions to any conclusions in my mind. Distance; distance and calm. Thinking logically, practically. Of course, there were any number of explanations—all that junk Rachel was always eating, all the crazy viruses going around, all the—well, other things: amebic dysentery. And in a small inner voice: amebic dysentery in the winter in Hillshire, New Jersey? Well, something. None of this was really thinking—my mind was rather empty, perhaps like a calm ocean out of which these sudden fish snouts poked.

The afternoon meeting went well. Naomi agreed to do the seating. Leaving, we stood in the door of the Community Center and looked up at the sky, which was snow-heavy and low. "What's the matter?" Naomi asked.

"What do you mean?"

"You weren't yourself."

"I thought I was very efficient."

"That you were." Naomi waited. We were in the car now, heading back to our neighborhood, and I was driving, considering answers, discarding them. The silence grew. "Let me know if I can do anything," she said as she got out at her house. The door slammed hard.

Now it was snowing. And suddenly I was incredibly tired. Just to sit here, sit and not move; let the snow obscure my sight through the windshield, pile up on the sides, higher and higher, bury the car. I shook myself and gunned the car up the hill, drove into the garage with a flourish. Goddamn dramatics!

Dr. Freeman called in the evening. "What's the matter?"

I reported carefully, also that Rachel's complaints had gone on for some time. I explained why I had ignored them. Then, in a rush, "Curt, I think she has ulcerative colitis."

"Nonsense!"

"Yes," I insisted. "The smell! It smells just the same as it used to with Sam."

He laughed. "Listen, lightning doesn't strike twice. Bloody stools all smell alike, and there can be dozens of other causes."

I listened. I listened and felt my stomach loosen up. But also felt numb as I considered what I had said. I must be crazy. Even to think a thing like that. It was this goddamn being alone; why was Mark always gone when something happened?

"Hey, are you there?" Dr. Freeman asked.

"Yes, of course." I thanked him for making me feel better; I would see him tomorrow. Then I took a sleeping pill.

In the morning Rachel felt sick, did not want to get out of bed, whined, "Can't Dr. Freeman come here?"

"What? When you don't even have a hundred five?" I was referring to the day we had left for the cruise on the S.S. *France* when I had taken her to his office with a hundred and five. He had given her a shot of penicillin and said, "Have a nice trip." That night she had eaten caviar.

Rachel refused to be amused. "I don't wanna."

"Come on," I wheedled. "You can wear the new garter belt." It was her first grown-up garment and went with a pair of crimson ribbed stockings. She succumbed to that lure.

Dr. Freeman examined her carefully; took blood, urine, and the stool sample we had brought. Then he said that he'd like to send her to a proctologist, since Dr. Zalinger was out of town. In answer to my anxious face he added, "He is an excellent man and right here in Hillshire." He looked up the number, dialed, spoke a few words, listened. Then, turning to me, "How old is Rachel now?"

"Nine." And suddenly, like an explosion in my head, yes, nine. Nine and three months. Sam had been nine and four months at the time of his first episode.

"You can go right over; he'll wait for you." Dr. Freeman wrote a name and address on his prescription pad.

But I just sat. Rachel was outside in the waiting room probably attempting another giant structure with the outsized Tinker Toys that were the office attraction. Each time we were there she'd try, but each time some toddler would walk into it and send it crashing. Last time she had laughed—not altogether amused—and said that it was like building a castle at the beach, trying to get it done before the big wave. "Listen," I said to Dr. Freeman. "Listen, Curt, could ulcerative colitis be genetic? Maybe something in Mark's and my genes—the combination, perhaps. I mean, Dan is healthy: he's from my first marriage. . . ."

Dr. Freeman was shaking his head; his pleasant face was stern. "I want you to stop this," he said. "I told you already, lightning doesn't strike twice."

"Okay." I got up, gathered my things. In the waiting room I found Rachel with a book. " No castles today?"

"I'm too tired."

I held her hand on the slippery snow outside, told her quickly about seeing another doctor. "A proctologist," I said. Oh, God, how to explain it to her.

But she asked, "Proctologist? Like in proctoscope? Will it hurt?"

"I don't think much." But wondered, how did she know? Driving slowly, carefully, I felt disoriented. *Never*, never would I have guessed that Sam had spoken to her about such matters. Yet how else could she know? Or had she overheard us? What else did she hear, know, sense? What else did she fear? I remembered how she had asked: do I have it?

Proctologists have a chair that is compatible with their particular examination. The patient kneels in it before takeoff. "More fun than a dentist's chair," the doctor said, and let Rachel operate some of the buttons and levers. He gave her time to get acquainted with the situation. When he proceeded to the examination, he let me hold her hand. It was quick. Alone in his office, he looked straight at me and said that he believed that Rachel had ulcerative colitis.

CHAPTER 5

FROM RACHEL'S POEM:
AT LAST, THE FOREST A CATHEDRAL

So my death is a lie!
I will live a lifetime,
not in a year, day, or moment.
In a lifetime.

MARCH 25, 1977

Back on full fluids, all the tubes are out, Rachel is corked. "Corked" means that the catheter which is sewn into her pouch is no longer attached to a tube or pump and is literally corked except when the pouch is being emptied and/or irrigated (by water squirted into it with a rubber syringe). This is the last step before this catheter will be removed altogether and normal intubation will begin. This intubation will be accomplished by insertion of a ten-inch plastic catheter into the nipple valve which keeps the pouch from leaking. In the beginning intubation will be done very frequently to keep the pouch from stretching too fast, but the final goal is that this built-in pouch requires no more emptying than the two or three times a day which are needed for an artificial appliance worn on the outside.

In the meantime Rachel is ambulatory and subject to all the jokes obviously provoked by a stiff piece of plastic tubing making a bulge under her nightgown. It is peculiar how funny these coarse and rather stupid comments seem. I presume because they connote a back-to-normal attitude; she is not too fragile to be teased. Though what is normal; how is normal? Is Rachel still Rachel? I mean, will Rachel healthy be the same as Rachel chronically ill? How much adjustment will there have to be? How much has she given up for health? Many unexplored vistas. I think I know the answers; I think she'll handle all this well. But still, who is to set standards for normal?

At the same time, everyone is pushing to get her home for Passover. It scares me. Is she ready? Well enough? I picture the glittering Seder table, the candles, the matzos, the endless ceremony. And I know we shall read *every* blessed word of the Haggadah— Rachel wouldn't allow a single deletion—and we shall argue about the ten plagues as usual, and I will get angry at Mark's naive apologia again. How tired she will get, sitting on her poor wounded butt. But apparently it is very important. To Dr. Gaon too. He had promised her way back in February that she would be home for the holidays. And in school May 1 to resume her research.

%   %   %

This narrative has become like an accordion, stretched out fifteen years to the yowl of the past, squeezed together for the moans of today. The middle chords were the incredible sounds of the night after the proctologist made his diagnosis.

Until the children were in bed, I was walking around well insulated in my Scarlett O'Hara thing: not now, not yet. It was essential that I first help Sam with his essay on the American Revolution; we incorporated a lot of the things we had learned in Williamsburg. Then I made brownies for Rachel and read her two stories and sang her all the long songs which I normally try to avoid. At last, though, they were asleep. Now was the time to call Paul.

St. Croix, the itinerary said. A bad connection, whistling and static, at last a soft voice. She would tell the doctor to call me back. Couldn't she call him to the telephone now? No, he was in a house at the beach, he had no telephone, he would get the message when he came up to the main house. "When?" I asked. "Perhaps tomorrow."

For a while then, I walked around. I was still under the influence of the calm of my actions; I had responded to the soft voice in St. Croix with equal gentleness. Really, I was rather amazing, the way I went on battle alert, the way I did not have hysterics, did not scare the kids. Sam had told me recently that all during his hospital stay he had never been afraid because I was always cheerful. "I figured, if something were wrong, you'd be a mess," he said. I had done that for him. Yes, I was a rock, the foundation on which my family rested, their stability.

Then in mid-thought, in mid-stride, right in the center of my bedroom, I sank down, folded myself up, stuck my fists against my mouth to muffle the cries. No, no, not Rachel; not my little girl. Not again. I can't stand it. I simply cannot bear it. I can't; I won't.

After a while I paced. Only to find, again and again, that I'd stand someplace, stand and stare, stand and fight down the rising hysteria, feeling it crest, then ebb. It was in my stomach, my gut; heat poured over me; ice chilled my feet. I crawled into bed, turned on the electric blanket and the heating pad, couldn't get warm, and then, in a terrible sweat, jumped up again and walked the floor some more.

At one o'clock the telephone rang. "Jean? Paul."

Thank God! Words poured out of me. On and on. Until I heard the silence. "Are you there?" I cried.

"I am here." After a while he could talk. In a hoarse voice. Perhaps the proctologist had made a mistake, don't get upset, we would see. Anyhow, Rachel could have a very minor case, nothing like Sam's; the range was tremendous. I listened to his voice, rather than the words. The voice of a friend, trying to find something to say that would be a comfort.

Later I pictured the scene. The tropical night, the moisture, the heavy smell of the red hibiscus. And Paul's bare feet on the sandy path up to the main house. Why had he gone there? For a bottle of club soda? For a can opener? Now he was walking back, and I had invaded his paradise. I knew the look on his face so well: concentration, a kind of stubbornness, an anger. How this disease obsessed him. I sat on my bed and cried for Paul, for Nina. Cried in guilt, then furiously—to hell with them, with all the fucking doctors; let them find an answer.

People speak of not closing an eye all night, Hackneyed phrase, but true on that occasion. Deep in the dark hours, awake and alert to all the demons in macabre dance, to all the knowledge of what was ahead, to the thoughts that would have to be blocked out in the morning so that I would be able to function. And the special horror because I had been there before. Oh, God, how could this happen again? My teeth in my fist, hating the drama and my dramatics.

At last the dark shapes that had lurked outside the windows throughout the night became our pine trees. Eerily beautiful, fat pillows of dense white snow bending the branches down to the ground, stark in the gray of almost-morning. Time for coffee, time to gather myself—Mark would be home this evening. Again an assault, a shock: Mark. And one more gush of angry tears.

Throughout Sam's illness Mark had been in more distress than I. Whether the reason for that was his extraordinary closeness to Sam or the quality in Mark that had made us decide long ago that it was he who was the Jewish Mother in the family. In any case, he was not able to achieve the kind of separation of which I was capable when I really needed it. Mark literally hurt with Sam.

Perhaps another explanation for my greater detachment was also that I was actually *doing* for the children each time they were ill. It was I who had the physical care, who did the chauffeuring to and from New York, the running up and down the stairs, the fetching of food, of medication. And I who dispensed comfort and reassurance and brought just one more glass of water. It was also I who took the assault, the front-line shock of dealing with the doctors, of receiving and interpreting the avalanche of information and, more important sometimes, the impressions of things left unsaid. Not to mention that it was I who was homogenizing the children's fears and furies, was trying to understand and ease the terrible ambivalences between their need of me and their anger because I could not really help them.

I suppose all this provided me with a sense of paying my dues; I did not need to bleed with them to attenuate the guilt. But Mark had none of the relief my labors gave me. Sometimes, during the really bad times, he had come home and we had actually treated him as a stranger. For hadn't he been gone while awful things had happened to Sam? Making me so damn hostile, there he was, waltzing in, saying, How are you? Like someone who expected a polite Fine, thank you.

It was one of the things we hadn't discussed—not so much because we were afraid of it as because it was nebulous, veiled, too wispy to touch. And there was the other aspect of the relationship: the solid love, and Sam's and Mark's likeness, their trust, and the fun they had together. But quite often I had seen Sam shield Mark quite deliberately from his empathetic pains; bad news was for Mommy.

Thinking of it that morning while making the coffee, I had a sense of dread. How would Rachel handle this? Theatrical, emphatic Rachel. Would she insist on extracting every last ounce of sympathy from her daddy? How could he tolerate that? Yet I cautioned myself not to regard him as a fragile creature: he had a different strength, a beautiful strength stemming from love; not my cerebral brand. And suddenly I couldn't wait for him to be back, to be there to talk to, to share the impossible burden. Hell, just to have him hold me.

The mug of coffee was marvelously comforting in my hand. Yes, I was feeling better. Perhaps because of the unusual indulgence of the night's orgy of suffering. Rachel, I thought, would have the immediate benefit of the right treatment. We did not have to go through the nightmare of searching for the right doctor—Paul's method of management would have every chance of success with her.

I told Mark as we were sitting in the car at Kennedy Airport. It was difficult for a moment because he still had his "foreign look." This was an alien quality I felt in him when he first returned after one of his trips, and it was a reaction we knew well. We had joked about it for years, probably for lack of other ways to handle it. Actually, it was so damn hard on me every time he left that I barricaded myself emotionally against him while he was gone. Then, when he returned, it took—as he had once put it so picturesquely—a blowtorch to melt the ice off me. That day again, I had to overcome the thought: Who is this foreign person? I had to force the words out. "Mark, Mark, I have something terrible to tell you."

He turned white, but said, "Wait!" and pulled me close. I buried my face against him, felt a crumbling inside; oh, safe; I could cry. He waited until I could talk, then said, "Tell me." And later we cried together. At last we had to start the motor; it had gotten terribly cold in the car. So we drove home.

Upon Paul's return, he put Rachel on a high dose of Prednisone immediately. There was no more talk of a minor case. It was an agony of repetition—the same bloody diarrhea, the same dreadful cramps, the same inability to eat. And again the child emerging from a siege on the toilet with curls soaked with perspiration and the muffled moans; she was as goddamn brave as her role model!

Fortunately, there was also the same prompt symptom relief from the Prednisone. But one difference: her face mooned almost instantly, since she had started off being a round-faced little girl and had not suffered Sam's original twenty-pound weight loss before being subjected to the medicine. When she started to look pretty bad, I offered to let her stay home, but she refused. Her social life, her activities, the play she was in—none of it could be missed. From the very beginning something was driving her to keep going. It made Sam angry; he couldn't understand why she would subject herself to the cruel comments that he was sure the kids were making about her appearance. Making the supreme sacrifice, he offered her the use of his trains, but she was too busy to accept.

So was he busy getting ready for his Bar Mitzvah. And I! The darn thing was growing into a Polish wedding, a Roman circus, a religious orgy. The Orthodox members of the family were coming for the whole weekend; they had to be housed and fed by our Orthodox friends. There would be an extended-family dinner in the synagogue's dining room on Friday night, a *kiddush* (a festive collation) for the whole congregation after the service on the Sabbath morning, and a giant dinner Saturday night in the banquet hall; the guest list had grown to over two hundred.

I was constantly torn between mirth and fury—how had this happened to me? Me, who'd always made fun of fancy Bar Mitzvahs. Me, who believed in the dictum never to invite anyone who didn't really want to come. I would neither have business acquaintances nor ever ever say, But we *must* have the Potamkins! However, it seemed to us that all our family and friends were so emotionally involved with Sam and us, with the very fact that Sam was alive and so much better, as well as with the thought that he'd have to face another round of surgery, that they wanted to share the moment with us, and we really wanted them there.

And the caterer did make elegant suggestions. He agreed with me that eight-course dinners were obscene, that green sherbet between soup and salad was gauche; in fact, we'd have salad instead of soup. As to the florist, well, he and I were creative together; the children's tables at the party would be in a simulated circus tent; it would be splendid. "Who needs this nonsense?" I yelled at Mark. God, we were emotional about that Bar Mitzvah.

Rachel was already on a reduced dose of Prednisone. We assured each other that the puffing was not really all that bad. Her dress had a dark rose velvet bodice and a pink organdy skirt. And my dress! Made for the occasion: ecru crepe, long-sleeved, slim. Mark, more concerned with the religious aspects, would wear striped trousers and morning coat to the service to give it full and formal respect. Both of us were brimming-eyed when we spoke of it. After all, we did have so much to be grateful for: Rachel was responding well, we had caught her disease in time, everything would be all right. If only Papa had lived to see . . . And my parents were coming from Chicago. And Sam had written this marvelous *droshe*, a personal explanation of what the portion he would read in the Torah meant to him. And Dan's future in-laws would be with us. Dan and Ruth would be getting married in July. A cornucopia of emotional events. "Are we nuts?" I asked Mark.

He shook his head, no. Mark is always less hung up about being corny.

Friday night. Uncle Shloime with the long beard cutting the *challa*; my parents finding all this orthodoxy weird, but being polite. Mark's Uncle Paul beaming because everything was as kosher as could be, plus as splendid as it had been back in Russia where Mark's family—very unstereotypically—had been rich. And *kreplach* in the soup and *tsimmes* with the pot roast and noodle kugel. Suddenly I noticed that the Bar Mitzvah boy was not at the table. I waited awhile, finally went to look for him, and found him in one of the back rows of the synagogue, sitting huddled in the knee-chest position, forehead streaming perspiration, white as a sheet. He was in dreadful pain. So while everyone else continued the festive meal, Mark and Sam and I drove into Manhattan. Paul, fortunately reached promptly on the telephone, had said that he would meet us at his office. Sam had an obstruction.

It is never entirely clear what the causes of obstructions are— they are not rare after extensive abdominal surgery and are blamed on adhesions, spontaneous kinks in the intestines, or foods improperly chewed. My own observation over the years makes me think that it is often a combination of these factors. Certainly, that night, it did not seem unreasonable to suppose that the excitement of the occasion had tensed Sam's insides enough to let some food get stuck. Paul proceeded on that assumption; put a tube down his throat and pumped him out. All the time we were perfectly certain that Sam would be in the hospital the next day, nor do I think that we really cared; it mattered only that he be out of danger, out of pain.

So there we were, Mark and I, in the waiting room, while Paul worked over Sam, trying not to hear the gagging, the choking sounds, and we tried desperately to squeeze some mileage out of our emergency humor. I painted fantasy situations about the festivities as they would evolve with the Bar Mitzvah boy absent; Mark smiled dutifully. However, at four A.M., a shaky but laughing Sam shook hands with Paul; said, "See you at nine in synagogue" and, deepening his voice to a stern note, "don't be late!"

"Late? Why would I be late after this good night's sleep?" Paul replied.

The tears shot into my eyes a few hours later when I saw Paul and Nina walk into the service; and if it was unbelievable that they were there, it was much more fantastic that we were, that Sam was. The synagogue was crowded. Aside from our guests, just about every member of the congregation had come that day. It gave me a feeling of love and support that was quite extraordinary. For me, the family's rebel in matters of religion, it was a revelation. So what that I could not believe in a Dear God who would make my children well, or in a bad one who had made them ill? I did believe in community, in belonging, in friendship. It was very moving. And belief or not, the fact that Sam was standing up there, was performing his functions perfectly, was a little miracle.

After the *amidah*—the silent worship—I hurried downstairs to look to the *kiddush*, but the caterer had things well in hand. Boiled salmon with parsley-stalk eyelashes winked from the tables, and each *gefilte fish* was festooned with a hard-boiled-egg daisy; it was too gorgeous for words. I heard the thundering herd of assorted guests and congregants approach. They grazed with amazing speed and concentration, and an hour later it was all over; even the decorations had been eaten. "Was everything all right, Madam?" the caterer asked; he was sweating. I said, oh, yes, and that I'd see him at night—even though the thought of another party and more food was terrible just then.

Outside, Mark put his arms around me. He held me a moment,

then said, "Like locusts!" But his voice shook. I replied that I had thought of buffalo. And was glad that he too was in control.

Just the same, the party was terrific that night. Short naps had restored us miraculously. Or perhaps some special adrenaline did the trick. In any case, it was wonderful and happy and we danced and danced and never had a sad thought. Only at the end of the meal, emptying the dregs in the wineglasses, when the festivities were almost over and Sam and Rachel chanted the after-dinner grace together, did I feel serious. Serious but not upset. Serious and incredibly happy because we had something that transcended our troubles. I looked over to where Mark was sitting and found his eyes waiting for me. And when Sam rose to make his speech, his parents held hands. Even in retrospect, it's hard to describe what we felt—certainly not the "aren't you proud of him?" jazz we were getting from everyone. Something quite other than pride: perhaps a sense of confidence, or even certainty, that Sam would be well. That Sam would be well in every sense.

The following weekend we checked him back into "Children's One." We were pleased that his former nurse, who had married in the interim, was going to take the eight-to-four shift again. She was still interested in jigsaw puzzles. We decided to do an abstract this time. It took the full six weeks of Sam's hospital stay to put it together.

Rachel was marvelous on this round. Even though she had her own troubles, suffering a flare-up on the day of Sam's surgery. She was shot back up to forty milligrams of Prednisone, and we began the weekly shuttle to Paul's office. And though she would cry in the car just before we got there and tell me that she hated Dr. Zalinger, that he hurt her, and why couldn't I come in with her and hold her hand, and please, please—in spite of that, she went through it all like a trooper. Not I, though. Destroyed, trying to disappear into the earlap chair in the waiting room, I would feel resentful of Paul for not allowing me with Rachel, for hurting her, for . . . oh, God, for not curing her already.

The routine was that Paul would have me called into his office when he had finished examining Rachel. There I'd find a well-composed child, asking intelligent questions, making charming jokes with him. Then, back in the car, more tears for me. By the time I got her home, I'd be a ball of tension, wanting to get back to New York and to the hospital and to Sam, also wanting to stay with her. But she made it easy. "Don't worry about me, Mom!" and she'd skip off. Or wave. "Give my love to Sam." Though once, in the rearview mirror, I saw her posture change into a slump after she thought me gone.

I'd drive off, impotent, impotent. And sometimes let go with some tears of my own.

April 2, 1977

After thirty-five days in the hospital, Rachel came home yesterday and is sitting in the kitchen with Ruth and Beth and me. She is scraping apples, mixing them with honey and ground hazelnuts, a bit of brown sugar, and sweet wine for the *haroseth* which we will need tonight at the Passover Seder. It's symbolic of the mortar the Children of Israel used when they laid bricks for the Egyptians; it represents their forced labor and their hardships. However, since it tastes delicious, we think of it as a treat, and we put a bit of it together with the maror, which is the symbol of bitterness and is made of pure horseradish.

Making the *haroseth* really scrumptious has been Rachel's specialty since she was a small girl. She shares the secret with her four-year-old niece now, whispering into Beth's ear. Beth nods seriously; she has both hands in the gook of soaked matzos and eggs and matzo meal that will make the dumplings. My daughter-in-law, Ruth, in the meantime, is crying over the horseradish, and Davey, because he is strong and six and the only man in the house right now, is helping our housekeeper, Caroline, to bring the heavy silver chest downstairs. Could I be happier?

What a move it was! To strip the hospital room, that very personal Rachel world. To take down the posters, pack the books; to cart off the forest—twelve plants, all flourishing; to shlep down the hair dryer, the hot pot, the suitcase with nightgowns and robes and slippers, the box with surgical supplies. Before leaving, before all the farewells from new but incredibly intense relationships, Rachel taught a young nurse who would take on her first pouch patient today how to insert the catheter to intubate the pouch. Then she wrote notes to everyone who was not right there to be thanked. And then we were at home and she was in her own bed, her face drawn and white. But so beautiful. The little kids are somewhat in awe, perhaps because of the fragile look of her hands; they didn't bounce on "Auntie Rachel's" bed as usual.

The *haroseth* finished, Rachel starts the nut torte, which is another tradition. It has stopped raining, and Davey and Beth have escaped into the garden, where they are chasing the dog. We laugh about their sudden courage: until last year they showed respect for the seven-pound Jaydee, but now that they own a dog twice his size, he does not awe them anymore. Also, they are four and six now, vastly more than a year older.

"Are you sure you're not too tired?" I ask Rachel, pointing at the batter; I'd be glad to take over.

"I'm tired, all right," she admits, but goes on pushing the dough off the bowl's sides with the rubber spatula.

And then we are talking about the fact that Sam came home from the hospital after the second surgery on Erev Pesach—the day before Passover—as well, and Rachel tells us that they had a big fight.

"I didn't know that," I say.

"I guess we were trying to establish ground rules. *I* was the patient now. I remember telling him that I was on twenty milligrams and he was on nothing. And he said yes, but his wound had to be irrigated."

"I didn't know that," I say again. I feel constricted, hurt, even though it was so long ago.

Ruth, who is very quiet but most observant, remarks practically and positively, with a lilt in her voice, "And now it's all over."

She is right, of course. The hurt feeling melts into a kind of hot butter sensation inside me. No, I could not be happier.

🌱 🌱 🌱

Just as she remembers, Rachel was down to twenty milligrams of Prednisone when Sam came home from the hospital the second time. Things were really going smoothly, and it was time to think of Dan's wedding in Boston. Looking back, I feel sorry that I did not enjoy this anticipation better, but I guess it was at that time that my reaction to the past year set in. It wasn't that I fell apart; it was only that I was devoured by so many anxieties—almost like a fear of the evil eye—and I felt that if I were to relax, to enjoy, to accept the idea that there was no immediate reason for concern, I'd be hit with another catastrophe. I can't even claim that this unease was based on realistic considerations, that I thought that the course of Rachel's illness would inevitably follow Sam's. No, I was quite convinced that she would benefit from the immediate and correct treatment she was getting. But what I was suffering from was a general pessimistic cast of mind, which is normally foreign to my nature.

And so the wedding. I wonder how much of an insult it was to my pride to see my two younger children in that wedding party. Sam, almost back to normal, already so mature with life knowledge, and Rachel, doing relatively well, but just the same a strange-looking little girl with her pouchy cheeks and fat neck in the beautiful long dress of mimosa yellow. Did anyone, did I, see her shining spirit, her courage? Did Dan? What had it been like for him in Ruth's world—a world already enough different from ours, a world in which people laughed, enjoyed their lives, their nice cars, their self-achieved luxuries? While we, heavy as flour paste, analytic, earnest, were always trying to deal with too much fear. Did Dan have to fight against a feeling that we were freaks? Of course none of this was verbalized, yet all of it caused terrible tension. Still, the wedding was happy. I watched Dan and Ruth dance, felt that things were good. Possibly, even, that he was well out of our lives. Expressing, perhaps, an unconscious wish of my own to escape.

However, a good summer in Hampton Bays did a lot to cure my "nerves." First of all, suddenly we saw Sam grow. Literally, stretch and grow, walk straight, swim and run at the beach and hit a nice tennis ball. His curls bleached by sun and ocean, the lean look of his shoulders I remembered from before the illness; he was obviously adjusting well to the ileostomy and did not require any kind of assistance from me anymore. There was no doubt that after the years of pain and dependence, after all the mental agony, the freedom which the surgery had restored to him was absolutely intoxicating.

Rachel too did well that summer, lost the look of the squirrel with hoarded nuts in its cheeks, and now that she approximated her old self, there was suddenly an avalanche of stories about how humiliating it had been to be so fat, so ugly. "Mommy, once I stayed in the girls' room all morning. The teacher thought I had cramps; I said I did, but it was because she'd sat Freddy next to me. He said, Yecch! when she said he had to sit there. It was humiliating."

However, she, as did we, presumed that her problems were now past, and so she drove the lifeguards insane with her sorties into any kind of ocean during that July and August. Twice she had to be fished out of the sea. Fortunately, I did not witness either incident and only had the report from one of the young men, who said modestly that it had been nothing much, only the current, you know. . . . Rachel, on the other hand, claimed that she could have gotten back by herself, "Easy!" and that it had been humiliating to be brought out of the water like a little kid. Just the same, she adored her savior, stood on her head before his high perch and wanted a two-piece swimsuit. In the fall, back home, she wrote him a letter, saying, "I fear that we will lose our friendship unless we communicate."

At school Rachel was expanding her life beyond the neighborhood. Lots of new friends. But also teachers who didn't bother to become involved. "You certainly are absent a lot!"

Tears. "He thinks I baby myself, that I'm not tough. I told you I should go! You made me stay home."

"Rachel, you could hardly stand. And you had a fever."

"Still. The kids laughed. And Beebee said he was right." Beebee was the special new friend, lanky, thin to the point of emaciation, at ten already elegant in the way fashion models are both stunning and ugly. With her came another "friend," Cheryl, a package deal. There were immediate complications. Beebee said that Cheryl was jealous of Rachel; she quoted her father, who was a psychiatrist, as saying that poor Cheryl was really quite sick, so possessive, and that he thought his daughter would be better off being best friends with Rachel, who was a very well-adjusted child in spite of being fat and having ulcerative colitis.

I watched with unease, saw the handwriting on the wall, tried to say gently that perhaps Beebee oughtn't to stay for sleep-overs quite so often. But, of course, it was hopeless. Sam, also watching, did not like Beebee at all. He said she ate like a wolf; I think he was jealous for Rachel, who had a tendency to gain weight just by looking at an Oreo. "And the way she talks to Rachel! Mom, she makes her cry."

But when I asked Rachel, she said that was dumb. Beebee was her best friend.

Sam was in a new school. It had not been easy for him to declare himself, to express a sentiment frowned upon by that part of his thirteen-year-old psyche which was still inhabited by the cowboy in him. However, the fact was that by the time he hit eighth grade he knew that he wanted a school with more challenge. And the Riverdale Country School challenged him, all right. Dan, who had also attended it, watched in amazement as Sam fell madly in love with everything—teachers, boys, even the crazy car pool from New Jersey to New York. One of the mothers was a notoriously poor driver which gave the boys cause for hilarity.

Early that first fall, when it was already flannel shirts and sweaters and windbreaker weather, Sam's class went for an extended outing into the wilds of New England, to provide the boys with the opportunity to experience nature in the raw. I understood that it would be pretty rough and suggested that Sam be excused. Mark agreed with me wholeheartedly. The boys were expected to test themselves on extended solos, equipped with nothing but a canteen of water and a pocketknife. Surely, we argued, it was too soon for Sam to be exposed to that much hardship. Yes, so we argued. But to no avail, especially since Paul sided with Sam: there was no physical reason for Sam not to go; as long as he had water, a deprivation of food would not hurt him. And of course, Paul said, psychologically it would be an invaluable experience. When he put it that way, I was suddenly rooting for it also, which gave Mark no choice but to join the bandwagon.

Of course, afterward we were glad that we had permitted him to go. Apparently the solo had been a very important experience. He had chosen to stay alone for twenty-four hours, and he had faced some demons in the lonely dark while he sat in his self-fashioned lean-to. He explained it to us shyly, saying that he thought of things he might never have considered under normal circumstances. Life is always so busy, he said, but up there it was very quiet.

I think perhaps that all this was especially significant for Sam, to whom self-sufficiency and privacy had been so long denied and who needed to prove himself most of all to himself. In the process he may have neglected receiving one of the benefits the school had expected him to derive—communing with nature. Asked about that by Mark, he shrugged. I guess listening to birdsong seemed like kid stuff compared with the bigger issues. And once returned from the solo, feeling himself wholeheartedly part of the bunch, he had enjoyed the rough camp life and the companionship of the other boys; he came home dirty and happy.

Normality! A terrible fight between Sam and Rachel while he

was running his bath; she wanted the tub first, to get ready for her T.V. program. Screams, Rachel hitting. I yanked them apart, sent them both to their rooms. The next thing I heard was Sam's scream. Rushing to the bathroom, seeing the tub steaming. Sam yelling, "She tried to scald me; she turned off the cold water!" Rachel, holding her belly, laughing, laughing. And one of Sam's rare rages, shaking her: "You idiot, you crazy idiot! What if . . ." impotent pause; then he belted her. And I in a rare pose of non-intervention, because boy, did she have it coming; and she, hurt, innocent: "It was a joke, a joke!" Tears, then makeup time. Both of them hung upside down from the chinning bars in the door-ways of their rooms. Rachel said, "I'm sorry, Sam."

"Okay."

Mark and I locked our doors: to hell with them; enough. Normality. Rachel was way down on the steroids; Paul spoke of remission.

Until December, when all hell broke loose. Suddenly Rachel was as ill as Sam had been. Yes, responding quickly to forty milligrams of Prednisone, but relapsing inevitably on the way down. Once at twenty mg, once at fifteen; once we got down as far as two and a half milligrams. That had been the worst time, because we had been so full of hope. Though really, it was hard to judge what was the "worst"—any one siege or the overall pattern that evolved. The look on Rachel's face when she had to start all over again, that first day of swallowing two pills four times a day. The steroidal red spots on her cheeks, and the way it revved up her motor so that she needed tranquilizers—half an Equanil in the morning and a whole one at night—but still she could not sleep. She asked us to leave the door open, to stay home, to be close; her demons took conventional forms—someone in the closet, under the bed, behind the curtain. Yet she was so darn plucky, laughed at herself, tried to be brave.

I guess for her the worst was the weight. She gained forty pounds in the next year, becoming square from round, and we faced the impossibility of finding clothes that fitted. That dreadful maroon gym suit in which she needed a size fourteen for her waist but which was miles too long; the ugly fashions in the "hefty," the "big girls," the "roly-poly" departments. Until we discovered Lane Bryant. I guess going there for the first time was traumatic only for me; Rachel was too young to have heard comedians refer to Lane Bryant Ladies. In fact, as far as Rachel was concerned, it was glorious—a whole floor of rack after rack of dresses, skirts, blouses, and even pants that fitted her, were proportioned to her size, were cute. I remember a light blue shift with white trim—we bought it short, because Rachel's legs were still slim and pretty, without the ugly striations Sam had had—the dress was a real success. On our first visit to Lane Bryant we went a little crazy; from then on Rachel had something her skinny girlfriends could envy: lots of new clothes.

Which made her less of an underdog, a fact Beebee didn't like one bit. The bloom was off that love affair. Another girl, Lonnie, had joined the circle; Rachel was being maneuvered into Cheryl's slot. However, and incomprehensible as it was for me, Rachel hung on. Beebee had told her that she had to understand that Lonnie was the ideal best friend because they had everything in common; Lonnie's father was a psychiatrist too. "Though my father says that Lonnie is very immature," Beebee added, leaving Rachel to hope for a change in fortune. Certainly there appeared to be something that Beebee needed from Rachel, especially from Rachel fat. It was painful to watch. I couldn't imagine why Rachel tolerated the girl's moodiness, the ups and downs, the quotes from the two shrink fathers now. She was being apprised that they had declared ulcerative colitis to be psychogenic and that Rachel's weight was not due to the steroids or the water accumulation they caused; it was due to self-hatred.

Sam was furious. "What's the matter with you?" he shouted at Rachel. "There she sits and stuffs herself with my whole Sara Lee banana cake while you chew on a carrot! And says junk about your weight. How can you be so dumb?"

Naturally, his anger did not help, because its basic premise— that Rachel was asking for it by exposing herself to anyone outside the family—was unacceptable to her. I told him to butt out, but could not take my own advice. What hung me up was to see her in her misery, to know that there wasn't a blessed thing I could do to help her with the pain, the indignities, the dangers of the disease. And on top of it to have to endure this abuse!

One day, when Rachel was in bed, hugely swollen and in great pain, I picked up the extension phone and heard her say, "Can't you come over afterwards?" Of course I should have hung up, but I listened to Beebee's reply. "No," she was saying. "No, I'm tired

of sitting at your house; it's boring. And all you want is pity."
Putting the receiver back carefully, Rachel's protest cut off, I was
shocked at my reaction of pure fury. For the rest of that day I
went around having imaginary arguments with Beebee King—how
unfair she had been, how gallantly Rachel was taking the whole
thing, the way she really had to be terribly ill before she missed a
day of school—oh, and I'd like to say a thing or two to that father
of hers as well. What the hell did he know about it, calling ulcerative colitis psychogenic? Obviously it was they who were crazy.
And cruel.

More and more I began to think that perhaps we should seek a
Dr. Chevalier for Rachel too. Mark questioned the advisability.
Did she need that kind of support or did I? A fair question. Certainly I realized that I wanted to share the burden, to be somewhat
released from the emotional stranglehold Rachel was having on
me. I felt uneasy about our lengthy discussions of Rachel's fears
and anxieties. Her increasing need for them; she would come to sit
at our bedside almost every night. Mark would long since have
fallen asleep while Rachel still talked and talked. How fat she was,
how ugly, Beebee's latest barb, and something mean a strange kid
had yelled after her. And how she hated to go to Paul for her
regular visits. "I'm just not living a normal life," she said one
night when my tiredness had made me push too hard for an end to
our talk. Trying to smile while feeling shocked and indignant
inside—those damn dramatics! But, God, how true. I answered,
"Come on, Rachel! I think you're doing pretty well. You manage
where others might just lie down and give in and be sick."

"Yes, but what if I don't make it?"

"What do you mean?"

"I mean if I have to have the operation after all? I could never
be as brave as Sam."

Heart constricting, I said, "Nonsense! But anyhow, there's no
question of the surgery; Paul said—"

She interrupted: "Dr. Zalinger didn't think Sam needed the
operation either."

"No, that's not true. When we came to Paul, Sam's illness had
already progressed very far. It's completely different with you; you
were started on the right treatment immediately."

"But what if—"

"Rachel, it's after midnight."

"But I am scared, Mommy."

I opened my covers, she came crawling in, I held her. Over and over, sometimes the same subject for weeks. And after the nightly hour, comforted, she'd let me tuck her into her own bed. Then I'd lie awake, tense, questioning my wisdom. Had I answered her constructively? Was I adding to her burdens with my own anxieties? Was I honest enough or too honest? And what were those strands that ran so persistently through these talks? Her fear of the operation, or a fear of doing less well than Sam?

She had said, "I could never stand it like Sam." What? The pain? The alteration? What had she, who seemed so oblivious in the early days of Sam's illness, observed that frightened her so much? Or was this simply sibling rivalry—a concern that Sam would always be number one, bravest in pain, triumphant in recovery? And why the heavy concentration on making *me* the arbiter, why was I so important, why did I have to be informed of each anxious thought when, basically, Rachel was an independent child? Perhaps it was because *my* anger—wherever the hell it sat in some submerged region of my mind—frightened her. Was she dumping on me to bribe (I love you, I need you) or to punish (suffer!) me?

Discussing it with Mark did not help. He understood my questions, he reassured me, he thought I was doing splendidly. Look at what I had been able to do for Sam, setting him free when he, Mark, might have been overprotective. No, I said, it had been different with Sam. Rachel was demanding something else. "She wants too much," I said lamely.

"Maybe you're just tired," Mark said gently. And "Let's ask Paul what he thinks about some supportive therapy for Rachel."

Paul was in favor. His orientation was that the state of the illness wrought inevitable psychological problems for the patient and the family and that some help was therefore a good idea. Informed that Rachel seemed concerned about following in Sam's footsteps, he said positively that we were now dealing with a different situation entirely. "Yes, I told her that," I said; but I privately thought that we were also dealing with a child now who did not look to him as her savior. It was pretty complex.

Rachel, when consulted, seemed intrigued. Perhaps because of all the stories about Beebee's and Lonnie's fathers, who, if nothing else, were colorful—allegedly they had said their daughters could smoke pot as long as they'd do it at home; imagine! Or maybe she was not going to miss anything of which Sam had partaken. In any case, she arrived cooperatively at the office of the woman doctor whom Dr. Chevalier had recommended. We went through the usual initial appointment for the three of us, then Rachel saw the doctor alone, and then Mark and I had a separate meeting with her. To me, the doctor seemed fine. Not young, with softly wrinkled cheeks and a high-pitched voice which was not shrill—like a gentle Eleanor Roosevelt, I thought. I liked her green office, the million plants and the way the light filtered through their foliage. I felt relieved to have Rachel in her care.

Maybe that was the trouble. Because Rachel began to put up a determined fight against continuing after only a couple of months. Her argument was that the visits took up too much of her time. Reminded that we had let her discontinue the six hours of Hebrew school per week in order to lighten the burden, she said yes, but she'd rather take oil painting. And having to see Dr. Zalinger every week was bad enough, and she hated pills, pills, pills. Pushed, she finally admitted that the doctor was icky, talked too sweetly, was too old, too ugly, and insisted on discussing Rachel's illness. "Mommy, she wants to talk of things I can only discuss with Daddy and you."

"Like what, love?"

"Like proctoscopies. And how I feel about them." And Rachel began to cry.

In the end it was Paul who made the decision to let her discontinue. He had talked it over with her and reached the understanding that she could quit provided that if he felt it wise at some later date, she would try once more with a different doctor. She came out of this conversation very much reassured; somehow she and Paul had been able to find a rapprochement. Driving home, she said to me that, after all, her case was very different from Sam's and she'd soon be much better and psychiatrists were really gross. "I mean, I can always talk to Paul if something bothers me," she said.

"Dr. Zalinger," I corrected.

"Yes, yes; I always call him Dr. Zalinger to his face. But I can think of him as Paul, can't I?"

"I suppose so," I replied uneasily. It had been Paul who had insisted that the children not slip into the familiar address.

So I cancelled Rachel's sessions with the psychiatrist, apologizing profusely, feeling guilty for Rachel about the "old and ugly" bit.

The doctor, however, remained untraumatized by the defection and wished Rachel and us good luck.

APRIL 4, 1977

I don't like the way Rachel looks. I didn't like the way she sat huddled at the Seder table; I think she is in pain, and I think she is running a fever. She says nonsense. The goddamn timetable.

Yes, she's right on the button; she has these next three weeks to regain her strength. Then she plans to return to Brown, move back into her room at the dorm, meet with all her professors. She hopes to arrange to make up her "incompletes" over the summer, and she will also finish the interviews with her patients to gather the data for her honors thesis. It's all set, with no provision for unforeseen events. At the end of the month Dan will come over from Boston and help her move out of the dormitory to her summer residence; she will be house-sitting for a professor who needs to have his fish fed and his avocado watered. A perfect setup, since she is not yet allowed to lift, carry, push, or pull anything heavy. But she will be able to swim and walk, and by the end of June she can play a quiet game of tennis. A quiet game of tennis for Rachel; that I have to see!

I am trying hard to determine whether my uneasy feeling is only anxiety, or whether my judgment that she is not doing well is correct. Not exactly a new predicament. Except, I had expected it to be forever past by now. Mark says patience. But he is watching her too.

Dan and Ruth and the children left today; Sam has gone back to his apartment. It is quiet in the house, four o'clock in the afternoon, Rachel is taking a nap. Perhaps that is all we need. Quiet and time.

❧ ❧ ❧

In the fall of 1967, when Rachel was almost eleven, she received an engraved invitation from the local dancing school. It requested the honor of teaching her the art and manners of ballroom dancing. Some years earlier, when the selfsame bid had been made for Sam's attendance, it had been a big joke around the house—Sam had had no inclination to be turned into a little gentleman, and even Mark and I had had to laugh at the very idea of Sam's asking a girl to dance. "And they make you check your guns before they let you into the saloon," Mark had warned Sam. Who had declared, "Forget it!"

It was a different matter now. Mark and I still thought that the formalities with which this class was conducted were quite hilarious, but Rachel had other ideas. Next to getting your period early, going to dancing school was the social pinnacle. And as luck had it, our name starting with B, Rachel received her bid before Beebee and Lonnie got theirs; their last names started with T's, another thing they had in common. During these intervening days, Beebee assured Rachel that she wouldn't be seen dead wearing white gloves and dancing with dumb boys who'd all be a head shorter than she, and what was more, she presumed that Rachel too would have the good sense not to make a fool of herself. "I mean, I don't want to hurt your feelings, but you know, the way you look!" However, once Beebee's invitation was received, it was another situation. Wailing loudly—through the open door I could hear every word in the next room—she declared that her idiot mother was making her go, did you ever hear of such a gross thing in your life, and please, please, would Rachel go too; she'd die if she'd have to go alone.

"What about Lonnie?" Rachel inquired cautiously.

"Her mother is making her go to a class in New York. It's where she went—Mrs. Tannenberg, I mean—and it's in French. That's even grosser."

"Poor Lonnie," Rachel said with glee.

"Yeah. Well, they are such snobs. Mrs. Tannenberg is related to the Gimbels."

"I'd rather be related to Saks Fifth." Rachel giggled at her own joke.

Beebee was on the floor, rolling and laughing. "Or to Lord Taylor."

"Very good. But did you know that we changed our name to Bergman from Bergdorf? My father didn't want to associate with the Bergdorf Goodmans anymore because they are in trade."

A successful afternoon.

The dress for dancing school was black velvet. One of the nice things about Lane Bryant was that the sizes sounded small. Since *everything* was for the fat, you could be a slim fat person and wear a size four. Rachel was very serious about this shopping trip. With great determination she tried on at least twenty different styles. I was getting weary, kept saying that this one looked very nice, yes, and this one too. But when we hit on the black, there was no question that it was far superior. "Terrific!" I gushed. She turned around and searched my eyes. Then said, "Do I look less fat in it?"

By the time the first lesson rolled around, I was enormously anxious. The whole venture seemed stupid to me. For once I agreed with Sam: why did Rachel have to expose herself to a bunch of kids in such a situation? I had given her plenty of ways out, but she had been steadfast in declaring that she had to go. "What do you mean: have to?" I had asked. She had given me an angry look and answered: because!

However, I must give the people who ran the school credit. The dancing master, fifty and sleek and with rosy cheeks, apparently sized up the situation immediately and kept choosing Rachel as his partner with whom he demonstrated the steps. And since Rachel had been born knowing how to dance, she was most graceful, and somehow it made her acceptable. Also, I suppose, those poor little boys might have been more comfortable with her than with some of the junior vamps who already sported pointy breasts and sinuous movements and tossed long hair. Excuse the sour grapes. One thing was sure, though: on Parents' Night I'd sit there stunned with admiration for Rachel. It would come to my mind the way I had first read the phrase "bizarre and even grotesque appearance," and the fear it had put into my heart. But here was Rachel, and she had somehow overcome.

Of course, not always. On some Thursdays she was not up to it.

On some Thursdays she was in bed with a fever. Perhaps just starting up on another increase in the steroids, which would make her legs hurt too much for her to walk. Or bleeding a lot. But those were the exceptional times. Most often Rachel went to school, to dancing, to oil painting, even to some parties; anything was possible as long as there weren't too many minutes between bathrooms. The only thing she missed out on totally was that lovely leisurely time-wasting—walking around town, sitting in a candy store over malteds, gossiping on street corners. Because, somehow, we always had to concoct interlocking time schedules that made it acceptable for me to be there with the car. Mothers were perfectly ordinary sights as chauffeurs; everyone's mother carpooled: it wasn't like being overprotective. Only Beebee caught on. "Your mother is always on top of us," she complained to Rachel.

Informed of which, I tried harder to be invisible.

CHAPTER 6

FROM RACHEL'S DIARY:

I got a sore throat at two o'clock today
and I sure hope it won't trigger another
attack because tomorrow is Lonnie's party
and on October 28 will be my sleep-over
birthday party. I will be twelve.

APRIL 15, 1977

Rachel is back in the hospital. Last Sunday, when she was running
a fever of a hundred and three and had pain, they checked her
back in. I think she was a little relieved; I certainly was. They
have started every kind of test; we are consulting infectious-disease
specialists and neurologists on top of the old team; they have
scanned her in the Department of Nuclear Medicine and will do a
spinal tap. There is talk of "checking out" everything from mono
to meningitis to massive infections to brain tumors. In the meantime, she has terrible headaches, and the fever keeps going up to a
hundred and five at night. The only thing that brings it down is a
special mattress which has coolants running through its plastic
veins. Turned on, it becomes icy; the patient lies on it and shakes
and shivers; but the fever drops. Not so different from the old-
fashioned cold bath, the alcohol rub; it appears to be more effective than all the medicines.

I don't know how she endures this too; I don't know how we do.
We put up "Hang In There, Baby!" again—how we identify with

the little cat with its beautiful, determined face—and we rein-stalled the plants and added a new poster of a girl by the ocean, a peaceful scene, serene and full of promise—soon, soon.

The part of Rachel that works best is the new pouch. It fills and empties satisfactorily; Rachel is on a schedule on which she has to intubate only every three hours during the day, and at night they are letting her sleep for four-hour stretches.

The rest? The doctors shrug, wear pained expressions, and some of them exhibit a veiled hostility toward Rachel. Like: what are you doing to baffle us? How they hate not knowing, not to be the conquering heroes. I feel a lot of anger toward some of them; I can taste their weekend impatience as every fiber strains to the golf course, the bright polo shirts, the striped pants. Meeting me in the hall—oh, especially the one young internist; I can almost see his eyes dart in an effort to escape seeing me, but as we meet face to face, the quick smile with full show of excellent teeth, the pat on my shoulder, the meaningless words. Coming into Rachel's room then, I blow: "Jackass!" Rachel laughs at me and defends him, says that his frustrations are enormous, that I am accusatory, that they are doing everything to find out. I feel shamed again that it is she who has to inject courage into me, suggest Scrabble, T.V., tapes, doing her hair, but really she is too tired. She sleeps a lot.

Dr. Gaon remains steadfastly our hero. Not only because the pouch is perfect, but because now, in this new nightmare, he can say, "I don't know."

❦ ❦ ❦

At the end of February 1968 Rachel started to write a diary. It was a red imitation-leather book with a gold key she kept carefully hidden. But every once in a while, she'd read me an excerpt. The day Paul had to shoot her back up to forty milligrams of Prednisone she read me the entry she had written on the previous day: "2/22/68: Things not going well with the u/c—down to 10 mg. Anticipate having to go up."

She always knew. And I would soon become apprised, because she would suggest seeing Dr. Zalinger even though there was no appointment scheduled. Normally she resented seeing him for the routine visits every other week, saying that she saw no reason to be subjected to a proctoscopy when she knew that everything was going well, that she would let us know if and when it was necessary to see him. And, indeed, she did know, and when the time came—

usually when she was coming down to the ten-milligram level of Prednisone—she would herself call him up. As on that morning. Hovering near her while she spoke to Paul, trying to listen and not to hear, I heard a pause during which Paul appeared to be questioning her. Then Rachel had said, "Yes, a lot of blood." And so I was driving her to his office.

To everyone's surprise, Rachel had turned out to be as stoic a patient as Sam had been; she had completely stopped permitting me to see her movements, and it was she who made the judgment that things were not going well. And sometimes, when I'd note the telltale signs of approaching trouble—the running to the bathroom, lack of appetite, a particular look of weariness, perhaps coupled with frantic activities as if she were trying to cram in fun and sports and work before being laid low again—and when my own anxiety mounted correspondingly, I'd eye the red diary on her shelf and wonder whether it was already noted there. "Loose stools and blood," perhaps? I never looked.

It may seem ridiculous or even irresponsible to an outsider that I did not feel that I had to monitor the symptoms of an eleven-year-old child's disease more closely; but I had a great feeling of conviction about her good sense and her need for as much autonomy as it was possible to give her to counteract her impotence regarding the disease. Once she had used the expression "I'm at his mercy" in connection with the unpleasantness of some examination and had said that Dr. Zalinger was insensitive to it. I had tried to explain that it was the illness which gave her the sense of being at its mercy. "I guess so," she had admitted, but I had not felt that I convinced her; Paul was too perfect a scapegoat. The difference between her and Sam was that Sam had met Paul when he had been almost at the end of the road, that for him Paul had been the last hope and finally the one who saved his life; for Rachel, he was the torturer. But *not* when she felt really ill. Not on this February morning. We were silent in the car as we approached his office.

That one was as bad as any exacerbation she had had in the two years of her illness. It kept Rachel out of school for four and a half months. By the time she could have gone back, the summer vacation had started. I remember that period primarily because it was the onset of her therapy with Dr. Klein. It was also a time of constant tension between the children. Sam, darling Sam, who had always protected Rachel around the neighborhood, had turned on her with a kind of vicious anger and disgust. Mark and I understood a little of it. It was clear, of course, that to Sam, Rachel's suffering was an unwelcome reminder of his own agonies which he was trying to forget or, certainly, to minimize. Coupled with that was the fact that she refused to take his advice and benefit from his experience.

What we could not see in him, or in ourselves, was the assault her looks were on all of us. I think that none of us could face the dreadful self-accusation that perhaps we were incapable of loving an ugly child. I began to have a glimmer of my own feelings only when, after Rachel had been in therapy awhile, she herself began to express her dislike of herself, the hatred of the offending body, her deep feeling about the ugliness. *And* the connection between ugly and bad. Another source of understanding came even years later when I read Gide's *Immoralist*, about the cured T.B. patient's feelings toward his wife, who is now stricken with the disease he communicated to her, who finds that she is blemished in his eyes. Defective goods.

As to Dr. Klein, I suppose the idea to try therapy again at that moment was born out of the terrific feeling of impotence the long exacerbation gave all of us, and the fact that Rachel certainly had the time to see someone now. Asked what she thought, Rachel shrugged and said yeah, she supposed this was an okay time to try it once more.

Dr. Klein came highly recommended by a Dr. Carlton. Dr. Carlton was a consulting psychiatrist to whom Paul had sent us; he was active in the infant National Foundation for Ileitis and Colitis, so that we could expect that his orientation toward the disease would be enlightened.

The experience of the visits with him was in itself interesting. Before our first encounter, he had required that I write him a history of Rachel's life—an undertaking that turned out to be pleasurable and reassuring for me. As I reread what I had written, laughed at some of my own humor, and smiled with love at some recollection, I suddenly, and for the length of a good moment, felt that we were an okay family.

Rachel liked Dr. Carlton a lot. She apparently felt free to discuss things with him that had been untrodden ground with the other therapist. It was therefore very disappointing to her that Dr. Carlton could not undertake her therapy himself. Explaining that it was not personal, that we had warned her from the beginning that Dr. Carlton was only a consultant, did not ease her sense of rejection. Which made Dr. Klein a poor second choice, but she did say that he was "Okay, I guess," and she liked the fact that he was in New Jersey. No more dragging into New York; when she was well enough, she could go to him without my assistance.

For all I knew then, they spent those first months playing gin rummy and telling jokes. I knew better than to probe; I was just glad that Rachel seemed satisfied to go. The only time I was made aware of Dr. Klein's skill in eliciting more than Rachel's shaggy-dog stories was when Paul made a caustic remark about him to Mark and me. Our subsequent questions were sidestepped with funny cracks—so much hostility can be hidden behind the usual shrink jokes—but later, on one of the periodic visits we had with Dr. Klein, we gathered that he had asked Paul to ease off on the proctoscopies.

It was a liberating breath of air for me to realize that the psychiatrist shared my indignation at the frequency of these examinations. Here, at last, someone was measuring the psychological damage these bodily invasions must wreak on a girl child against their scientific value. I had long, though silently, sided with Rachel when she had protested against the necessity of routine "scopes"; there was no goddamn reason, she said, for those periodic "looks." Secretly I considered Paul's insistence on the necessity for exact knowledge, for measuring the condition to the nth degree, obsessive. I raved to Mark, "Let him do his research on mice."

Mark was torn too. On Paul's urging, he had just gotten involved in that brand-new organization which called itself, grandiosely, the National Foundation for Ileitis and Colitis, Inc. Its purpose was to raise money for reasearch to find the cause and cure of these diseases; to gain political clout to get a slice of the health money from Washington; to disseminate knowledge about the diseases and the differences between them: ulcerative colitis, which affected the colon and could therefore be surgically cured by a proctocolectomy; and ileitis and Crohn's disease, or granulomatous colitis—diseases affecting both the colon and the ileum which, because one couldn't live without an ileum, were potentially not curable at all. Such basic knowledge was the Foundation's goal, as well as information about research, treatments, findings to be dispensed to doctors and laymen both. Not least of all: to give sufferers a central place to which they could come for information and help. A grand design. The Foundation had been started by a young lawyer whose wife suffered from ileitis. Mark was determined to put his efforts into it as well. Okay, so how can you stand in the way of research?

"I don't want to stand in its way; I just don't want Rachel harmed."

"It's not going to harm her; she's not such a delicate plant. After all, Sam tolerated it too."

"That was different."

"How?"

"Because it's an invasion, and because she's a girl."

Mark laughed. "That from you. The double standard, no less." I knew he was trying to tease me, to change the mood, the subject; he hated it when I was critical of Paul. But I didn't feel like being humored. I said crossly, "Look, it isn't *lèse majesté* if I don't agree with every last thing Paul does. You know what I think of him, but this business of 'scoping' a preadolescent girl routinely is poor judgment. He ought to listen to Dr. Klein. In fact, he ought to listen to Rachel."

"He can't let Rachel—or her psychiatrist, for that matter—dictate to him how to practice medicine."

"I don't know why not, unless it's an ego thing." I raised my voice; I was getting angry. "And that's what it is! God forbid someone tells God what to do! It so happens that I see nothing wrong in a doctor listening to a patient; it's Rachel who knows how much pain or blood she has. If she tells him that there is an improvement, he can take her word for it."

"She isn't twelve yet."

"So what? She is intelligent and she's reliable."

Mark shrugged. In the silence that followed, I tried to calm myself, tried not to go on into another useless diatribe. It was stupid to get so emotional. Basically, Mark and I did not disagree; it was only his dislike of facing the ambivalence of our feelings for Paul. Of course we loved him—personally because he was warm and bright and caring and because of a quality of honesty he possessed that was almost naive and very appealing. As to our medical opinion about him, there was not a day when we didn't talk of the fact that it had been his judgment, his timing that had scheduled Sam's surgery at the exact right moment. We would look at Sam, see him shoot up and come into his own, and we felt that every credit was due Paul. But! And that "but" was hard for both of us to accept. Though I was able to intellectualize it; I could say, Of course we also resent and fear and distrust him because he couldn't save Sam from the surgery, and because he isn't curing Rachel, but mostly because we need him so damn much! It wasn't easy to deal with.

Of course, I had a terrific outlet for many of my frustrations now. I had stopped writing poetry and was doing short stories. It was a great relief, because all the difficult emotions could now be used in satire or pathos or nice straight prose without being destructive. I wrote a story called "Filet Mignon on Thursday," which at last permitted me to deal with the guilt feelings that Sam and I had accumulated when we had moved him from the ward to "Children's One." It was a veritable paradise of spillage! Except for the rejection slips that kept stuffing up the mailbox. I framed the first one from *The New Yorker*, but soon they were no longer amusing.

Then, by the time the first acceptance arrived, Rachel and I went a little crazy. It was on a gloomy day while she was in bed and I disheartened—each day got longer and longer, and the hematology project she was doing as an independent study to fill her time was already over fifty pages in length, not to mention the two sketch pads of drawings and diagrams. It was somehow terribly depressing. I went downstairs to get the mail and returned to sit on the side of her bed to open it. A couple of get-well cards to add to her collection, and then I opened an envelope to find a green check fluttering out. Sixty dollars for "Mrs. Dearfield's Thunderstorm"! Rachel and I did a wild Indian dance, finally sobered enough to look to see which magazine had accepted it. Something called *Mr.*

"Never heard of it," said Rachel.

"Me neither."

"But you sent it to them."

"Well, you know how I do it." I had a method. From a copy of *Writer's Market* I had picked ten publications in each category. Love stories to go to the popular mags, sexy ones to the men's trade, those I considered highbrow to the little mags, the Jewish ones to *Hadassah*, and so on. Of course, later I found out that all this was nonsense. Jewish subjects invariably ended up in a Catholic publication, and why a particular story was bought and by whom remained a mystery. In fact, some of my very most serious stories ended up in the confessionals after I lost patience and, half as a joke and half in an effort to finally make some money, converted them to that genre. The humiliating thing was how minor the necessary changes were!

Anyhow, that morning I set out to find a *Mr.* The man at the store where I usually buy magazines said reproachfully, "Mrs. Bergman, you know I don't carry that stuff." And the man at the place where I found a copy offered me a brown paper bag. The children thought it was marvelous, but I was quite uneasy, insisted on using a pen name, and mainly appreciated it all as a diversion in those weeks of gloom. None of us ever figured out why the editor had bought my story, which, while it dealt with a lady who had an affair with a lifeguard, was rather mild stuff in that setting. When Mrs. Dearfield finally arrived in print, Mark said that she was like a daisy on a compost heap. Fortunately, the following month brought an acceptance note from *Transatlantic Review*, and I felt my dignity restored and could finally see my name in print.

In addition to her other woes, Rachel began to suffer from headaches at that time. Only she called them "sinus aches" and would hold the bridge of her nose with three fingers, indicating where it hurt. She would also develop an almost transparent pallor and purplish bruises under her eyes, so that I knew that she was in a lot of discomfort. We made an appointment to check out her sinuses with an ear, nose, and throat specialist, who, on hearing that she suffered from ulcerative colitis, kept his examination to a slipshod minimum. It was another encounter with a physician who regarded the term "ulcerative colitis patient" as a synonym for "certified nut"—her headaches must be psychosomatic! Fortunately, they did get better after Paul took her off the Azulfidine, a drug effective with some ulcerative colitis sufferers which, however, had not been helpful to Sam or, apparently, to Rachel. Then, when we appoached the dreaded twenty-milligram line of the journey off the Prednisone, passed that landmark, went down to ten and finally to five, and still there was no relapse, we suddenly noticed that it was summer, that school was over, that it was time to move to the shore.

The difference between not going to school because of illness and not going because of vacation is profound. One is a terrible deprivation, the other pure joy. This was the first year in which we had rented a house closer to the tennis club in Quogue, and suddenly I found that I was actually sitting on the lawn in front of the house, looking out over a lovely, peaceful pond which, at its far end, abutted the beach and ocean. A combined view of bucolic farmland and seascape. Foam leaping to the horizon and cows grazing across the creek, and the reason why I was sitting so blissfully was that Sam and Rachel had taken their bikes to the club.

I was like a normal mother of kids that age; I had some leisure; I had peace of mind. In fact, I had no excuse to keep me from finally starting the novel that had been knocking around my head for years, the novel I was going to write "someday!" Later during the day I might go down to the club myself for a game of tennis, and there I would see and wave to my kids. Sam had made friends with a terrific man named Mike. He had a gray beard and a most beautiful body and a history of having rebuilt his life and health by physical exercise (and a new wife, I suspect!). In any case, he had taken Sam in hand. They were running and swimming and playing tennis and tossing a ridiculous medicine ball around; I couldn't lift it, it was so heavy. Sam was in heaven.

As to Rachel, she was the tennis whiz, beating most of the women and all the girls. Red Corning, who was the pro that year, trained her hard. Once, watching, I saw him chase her around unmercifully yelling, "Run, goddamn it, run!" Until, at the end, she broke into exhausted tears. That evening Red came for drinks, and Rachel offered to take him sailing in the little Sailfish we had gotten. A half hour later Mark lent Red dry clothes. It was an accident, though Rachel was dry. "He just slid off," she said with regretful mien. She was a very good sailor as well as tennis player. And lost twenty of her forty steroid pounds that summer.

On our return from the country, we participated in a research study. Paul had put us in touch with a California woman who wanted to interview us as a family. The purpose of the study was to investigate sociopsychological data on families in which more than one member was stricken with ulcerative colitis, and apparently there were legions. We were by no means that solitary elm struck twice by lightning. I smiled ruefully, remembering Dr. Freeman's remark—had it been less than three years ago?

Mark, Rachel, Sam, and I, dressed nicely, each of us with individual expectations and anxieties. I suppose my concern was to convince the researcher of our terrific adjustment, to nix the rumor that family pressure produced ulcerative colitis in children; in short, to lay my ghosts to rest. Sure, I'd cooperate; sure, I might have to reveal that while we did not pressure our children for grades, Mark did have this unfortunate joke—any child who came home with an A would be asked why he had not gotten an A-plus. And Mark? On the drive to Mt. Sinai Hospital, where the meeting was to be held, he spoke little, smoked his pipe, wore a sports jacket, and altogether presented the picture of a relaxed country squire somewhat unlike himself except in rare vacation moments. It had made me smile. He too was preparing to tip the investigation to results he expected. But it was Sam who was uncharacteristically open about his feelings. He was looking forward to the interview. He would tell them, he really would; he would explain that it was ridiculous to suffer from this disease when one could be well after the surgery. He would tell them that only creeps let themselves be handicapped, that there was no reason not to participate in sports. . . .

Arrived, we were put into a small office, and after a while a pleasant woman had greeted us and had then invited Rachel into another room. Two hours later, she asked Sam and Mark and me to join them. The next thirty minutes were spent answering questions about family routine. Which meals did we eat together, did the children have separate rooms, how many cars did we own, what T.V. shows were the kids watching and did we restrict their T.V. viewing? More socio than psycho, I thought, and expected that the next step in the procedure would be private interviews—hopefully, not long ones such as Rachel's had been, since it was already close to five o'clock. But no, our interrogator rose presently, shook hands with all of us, thanked us, wished Rachel good luck, and saw us out. All the while Sam's indignation had risen visibly, and I only hoped that he would contain it until we were out of her hearing. He barely made it before exploding about how dumb the questions were, what he thought of witless ladies who spent their lives asking questions from a prepared questionnaire and writing down the answers—any census taker could do that—and what was more, the queries hadn't been to the point. In a family in which two children had ulcerative colitis, how come only the younger one was interviewed when the older obviously knew more? Here Rachel, who had been listening with a satisfied smile, interrupted to say that she knew why.

"Well?" Sam challenged.

"Because you don't have ulcerative colitis anymore. I'm the only one in the family who is sick."

"But I know what it's like. I have much more experience—"

"But now you're only part of the family picture of the patient," Rachel quoted.

We had come to the car, the kids jostled each other getting in, Rachel yelled that Sam was hurting her. Mark told them to pipe down. Then there was silence. Feeling my own sense of letdown, I could understand Sam's frustration. But at last it was Mark who put it in perspective for us. "Sam," he said, "we let our imaginations run away with us. I think we all thought we could contribute something. It's always painful when no one appreciates the pearls you want to bestow." He smiled around his pipestem; I felt suddenly delighted with him. Mark, who sometimes acted so dense on psychological matters, but whose instincts were always so good! But Sam was not ready to yield. "We *do* have something to contribute, we *do* have experience. What is this dumb survey all about, anyhow?"

"I guess we'll see it one day when it is compiled."

"Sociological crap," Sam predicted.

I tended to agree with him.

Discussing the incident when we were alone, Mark and I spoke of how weird it had been. How all of us—except perhaps Rachel, who was the patient—had a vested interest. Guilt? Or egotism?

When a fresh exacerbation broke out in October, Paul decided to try enemas containing fifty milligrams of cortisone. He promised Rachel that administering the steroid in this fashion would not moon her. But unfortunately, it was soon apparent that it did not help either. Nor was Rachel able to tolerate high steroids this time; sugar had been found in her urine, one of the always dreaded complications: a steroid-induced diabetes. We had come to the end of a road. Of course, we knew that it was a moment of crisis, though again, as with Sam, I simply did not permit my mind to turn to the possibility of surgery. Paul would think of something. And apparently he had. He wanted Mark and me to go to see Dr. Jacob Dash, a hematologist, to have him explain all about an immunosuppressive drug they were thinking of using on Rachel. "I want Jake to tell you about it; it's really his field. We are working on this together, but I think it's best if you ask him all your questions." Of course, we understood Paul's fine point—he was eliminating the element of automatic trust in a friend; he didn't want us to make a decision "because Paul said so." Nor did he want to restrain us from pestering the doctor with a million questions. Our appointment was for the following week.

In the meantime there was Rachel's twelfth birthday. The planned sleep-over party had to be cancelled because the innocuous sore throat about which Rachel had worried in her diary had, indeed, led to the present attack. We amused ourselves by making out rain checks (real bank checks on which we had painted ducks in slickers) guaranteeing to the guests that the party would take place one sunny day. That kept us busy and laughing for a day. And then I could buy presents—far too many presents—to compensate. A robe with matching pajamas, dresses, sweaters, a new tennis racquet, and a ring with a little gold rose on top. Rachel fake-served an ace into the living room and said fervently, "How I love tennis!" She laid the racket back on the birthday table. From a habit dating back to my childhood, birthday tables were adorned with a burning candle when first viewed. It had to be blown out with a wish. Oh, Lord! Would she ever be able to wish for something ordinary? For a boy to kiss her, for a good mark on a test, for me not to find out that she had broken my good vase? At this point, I knew, a wish was too important to waste on the mundane. We all closed our eyes while she blew.

Mark and I were reflective on our way to Dr. Dash's office. We spoke of the advance in knowledge about inflammatory bowel diseases that had been achieved in the recent past. Or was it only that *we* knew so much more from our own experience and from Mark's involvement at the Foundation? No, we decided. There was more to know.

And now we had to make another decision. With some irony I said that I found it harder and harder to rely on my wisdom. "It seems to me that there's a pile of psychological evidence that half the time my motivations are not what I think they are. So how can I decide? *What is best?*"

"Best!" Mark said bitterly. "You mean, the least of the evils!"

From Paul we knew that the drug in question was called 6-mercaptopurine—6-MP for short; trade name: Purinethol. It was an immunosuppressive agent. Paul had suggested that we must have heard it mentioned in connection with kidney transplants where it was administered to prevent rejection. As far as we understood, ulcerative colitis might also be influenced by a kind of autoimmunity. "Do you understand what he meant?" I asked Mark.

"I'm not sure. I guess they think that ulcerative colitis could be caused by the patients' self-allergies."

"Self-allergies?"

"The phrase Paul used was that ulcerative colitis might be a disease autoimmune in origin. I guess that means being allergic to something in your own tissues."

"I guess." I was reading the numbers along Park Avenue, searching for Dr. Dash's office. I said, "Well, maybe we'll know more after our appointment." And then, "There, quick! Someone is pulling out right in front of the house."

Paul had told us that we would like Dr. Dash. He had been right. He was tall, dark, soft-spoken. But leaving his office a couple of hours later, we did not understand the philosophy behind the medical theory much better than we had from our discussions with Paul. However, Dr. Dash had alleviated our fears of the drug considerably by assuring us that Rachel's blood would be constantly monitored so that any bad effect would be noticed in plenty of time to be reversed. He spoke of the fact that while the application of 6-MP to ulcerative colitis was fairly innovative and still experimental, the drug itself had been amply tested in other uses. Again and again, he used the phrase "Completely reversible!" Giving me a moment of *déja vù*; making me remember the way we had been when we made the decision to let Paul manage Sam on the high steroids. Yes, the bad effects Sam had suffered from the steroids had proved to be reversible, with the exception of the striations on his legs, which had, however, faded and were no longer visible now that Sam was getting to be hairy. Suddenly I heard Mark say, "Exactly what is the danger we are talking about? Are you talking of leukemia?"

Dr. Dash met his look. "No."

"But there are other dangerous blood diseases?"

"Yes. There is a danger of bone-marrow depression. There could also be initial nausea and vomiting, though that is usually transient. And infection is theoretically a possibility, due to impaired immune response expected from the treatment, as well as leukopenia which may result from bone-marrow depression. But look . . ." Dr. Dash raised his hands in a gesture that was not quite a supplication; his face had reddened. "Look," he said, "the dangers that exist can be avoided. If there are the slightest signs, we shall discontinue the treatment immediately."

It was a moment fraught with emotion. I knew what Mark would ask next, and it made me cringe. Yet I wanted him to ask it. And he did. "If it were your child, would you include her in this experiment?"

Jake Dash said that he would. We believed him.

It was not a new experience for me; I reacted typically. On leaving Dr. Dash's office, I felt mellow with gratitude, confidence— nay, belief. But with each passing mile, the doubts returned, and the anger. "Wouldn't it be a hell of a lot better if the precious Foundation would first undertake a research project on the use of six-MP in ulcerative colitis?" And minutes later, "In the end I know they'll find the answer in genetics." Two kids, both nine years old at onset; it couldn't be a coincidence. And, "What the hell is leukopenia?" Mark let me spill it out. When we were almost home, he asked, "Do we have a choice?"

That stopped me. Yes, did we have a choice? The heavy application of Prednisone was out, because of the sugar in Rachel's urine. The cortisone enemas had not worked. Azulfidine was not doing the trick and was giving her the headaches. Surgery? When there was something new to try? Something not dangerous if carefully watched? We really had no choice; we had to try it. But I said, still angrily, "At least let's get another opinion. Zalinger and Dash are probably writing a paper on this right now!" God, how I hated for Rachel to be their guinea pig.

"Okay. Tomorrow I'll find out who is the best man in this field."

And so we flew to the Mayo Clinic to see the famous Dr. Bernard Baldwin. He was a man who had published countless articles and who was considered an outstanding authority; he had experimented with the 6-MP for a longer time than any other researcher. After examining Rachel, he readily endorsed the use of it in her case. On viewing Rachel's x-rays which we had brought along, he made a remark that burned itself into Mark's and my consciousness like a branding iron. Standing before the lit panel, he nodded his head and said, "Yes, yes indeed, I would definitely recommend using the six-mercaptopurine. It has proved to be very effective in cases of granulomatous inflammations."

Only on the plane going back, with Rachel settled across the aisle playing gin rummy with an elderly gentleman, could we talk of it. "Granulomatous! That means Crohn's disease?" Mark asked.

"I think so." Which meant that the ileum as well as the colon was involved—the ileum, without which one could not live. It also meant that there was no cure, that even the removal of the dispensable colon could not bring about a total solution. People with Crohn's disease had many operations without permanent cures. We had heard about a woman who had been operated on fourteen times. "Paul lied to us," I said, and began to cry.

Rachel was laughing loudly. She called over to us, "I won; I schneidered him."

I wiped my eyes, said hastily that she wasn't to pressure the gentleman for another game. He assured me that he was having fun, said to Rachel, "Come on, your deal."

I turned back to Mark. He spoke tightly: "Don't jump to conclusions; we'll see Paul tomorrow."

But sitting across from Paul the next day, listening to Mark report on the consultation, watching Paul's face—the intensity, the interest, the concern—I felt so betrayed that I had a sensation of being gutted with hatred. I am empty, burned out, and all the debris would ooze out of me if I opened my mouth. I clenched my teeth—Paul too. They, all of them . . . Yet, suddenly, I was speaking, interrupting: "Why did you lie to us?" My voice was okay, only hoarse.

Both Mark and Paul turned to me. "Lie to you?" Paul asked.

Mark made a gesture of erasing my words.

"Yes, lie. Dr. Baldwin said Rachel has the granu . . . the granulo . . ." I couldn't get the word straight.

"Granulomatous?" Paul asked.

"Yes, that type."

"I didn't lie to you. Rachel does not have granulomatous colitis," Paul said firmly.

We all sat back in our chairs and stared at each other. The heat in my stomach was a red sun. My feet were tingling.

"Are you sure?" Mark asked.

Paul sat forward, hit the desk. "You misunderstood Baldwin."

"How can you be absolutely sure?" Mark repeated.

"Because I can read that x-ray."

"Better than the famous man at Mayo?" Hating how snide I sounded, when really inside I was beginning to breathe, to live. . . .

"Yes. No. You must have gotten things mixed up."

We looked at each other some more. Then Paul said again, "You must have misunderstood him."

"Okay," Mark agreed. He reached over and took my hand. His was hot. But I was also warming up, the heat from my stomach spreading out, coursing through, delicious. Oh, God, thank God. I laughed out loud. But did not explain. To be so glad that Rachel had only ulcerative colitis!

When we kissed good-bye, I hugged Paul for apology. He hugged me back.

At first they tested Rachel's blood every week, but when her counts remained normal while they were trying to establish the right dosage, she had to have it checked only every other week, then every third. All kinds of combinations were attempted: very small amounts of Prednisone, some Azulfidine, some Cantil in combination with the 6-MP, which was tried on a three pills (of fifty milligrams each) per day basis; then later it steadied down to one a day alternating with two on the following day. There was no dramatic improvement, unless we considered the fact that she was on much less steroid a step in the right direction. And the tape with which we continued to test her urine stopped turning the green that indicated diabetes. Not to mention that she was going to school regularly. And now that she had access to a hematologist, the independent project on hematology which she had started originally to occupy her time and mind during her confinement really blossomed, and we had become involved in it ourselves. Dr. Dash lent her books; we all pored over them, trying to understand the lingo because now we were suddenly terribly interested in blood; in immunology; in reds, whites, and platelets.

Dr. Dash became Rachel's favorite doctor. As she put it only semihumorously, "His pinpricks in the finger compare favorably with proctoscopies!" And of course, her visits with Dr. Dash were pleasant; they discussed Rachel's project, Dr. Dash's children, skating, and the fact that Sam was playing ice hockey against all doctor's orders. While the appointments with Paul were associated with pain and embarrassment. Not to mention the ordeal involved when new x-rays had to be taken. Apparently the most painful part of this procedure was the infusion of air required for better diagnostic viewing. Rachel was truly terrified of that.

I was also unhappy about her school. Some of the progressive ways were resulting not in the freedom we had anticipated but in outright chaos. I witnessed a math class one day and was appalled at the noise. The idea was that each child was working at its own speed, but the result was a constant clamor for the teacher. "I'm stuck, Mr. Jones!" "I can't do it!" "Me next!" And the poor man hurrying from child to child. Rachel somehow wriggled through. Tests could be taken at the child's convenience at the end of each section, and she seemed to survive from section to section. But she was always complaining that she didn't know what she was doing, and how was she ever to get into medical school if she didn't have basic math?

Looking back, it's hard to say what persuaded me to start campaigning for a change of school: the turmoil or the math? Yes, I wanted Rachel in a "nice" environment, and I did think that a more structured situation would result in better working conditions. But it also entered into my consideration that she ought to have fewer emotional frustrations. When I first suggested the switch, though, I ran smack into the reverse snobbism of public versus private school. Rachel said she would not go to that idiot school and wear nice little plaid skirts and gray blazers and have kids on the street know that she went to a private school. It was a little difficult to argue, considering that originally we had moved to New Jersey to escape the necessity of private schooling in New York. And now I was urging the last of my chicks to abandon the democratic ideal.

Whatever scruples I felt, and whatever objections Rachel had, melted during a pleasant interview at the proposed new school. I knew that Rachel liked what she heard about the educational methods, and she liked the grounds, the tennis courts, the orderly atmosphere. I think in an unconscious way she was plain tired of always having to fight: the disease, the situation with Beebee, the commotion in class. Walking home—the school was only a few blocks from our house—Rachel said, well, she wouldn't get in anyhow, not with her math! There had been a roomful of applicants taking the entrance examination, and there were only three open places on her grade level. I said that we would see.

By the time the letter of acceptance came in May, she was happy to go. And it came just in time to afford a moment of pleasure during a very bad period when Rachel almost landed in the hospital. In spite of the 6-MP, Paul had to jack her up to sixty milligrams of something called Celestone, a different type of cortisone which, it was hoped, would not mess up her blood sugar again.

The deal we made with Paul in order to avoid hospitalization was that I would bring Rachel down to his office every day. When the worst of the bleeding had stopped, she said to me, "I guess the cortisone is a necessary evil."

That summer Rachel lost all the steroid weight. Throughout the years of her illness, whenever she had to be on high doses, her main concern—once she was out of the initial period of terrible pain—had been the weight. Paul would promise to get her off the drugs as quickly as possible, but we knew that once she had an exacerbation it would be a good four months until she could be taken off steroids. And everyone, including the doctors, assumed that the weight which had been manufactured by the water retention due to the medication would simply melt away once the patient was off its cause. Rachel had found that this was not so. The weight was solid, had to be dieted off; and in Rachel's case, to lose weight meant near-starvation. I was terribly torn: on one hand, absolutely sympathetic to her desire to be slim; on the other, scared to permit a diet that to me spelled malnutrition. I had very little power to interfere. Rachel, perhaps with the prospect of the new school, the new start, was determined.

As to the doctors—Paul as well as Dr. Klein—they frankly did not believe me. The attitude was that fond Jewish mothers always want to stuff their darlings unreasonably. I remember a session when Mark, who was also very much worried, tried to convince Dr. Klein that Rachel was living on watermelon and coffee. Dr. Klein smiled and said that adolescent girls quite frequently cheat on their diets. Looking at that smile, smug in its superior knowledge, I knew that there was nothing I could do to convince him.

Nor was there a way for us to agree on the nature of Rachel's disease. Our observation over the years with both Rachel and Sam had been that the trigger for an exacerbation was most often a cold or some other kind of minor physical ailment. Dr. Klein, however, tied each incident to one of Mark's business trips. Part of the reason I thought him so wrong was the fact that the trips were mostly short. And since Mark worked crazy hours anyhow, it wasn't all that unusual for the kids not to see him for a few days even when he was in town. Additionally, whenever he took off I became a real Supermother. This was due to my own childhood trauma during my father's business trips; my mother had reacted very poorly to being left, and I wasn't about to repeat her mistakes. So I could not, even on careful analysis, detect any kind of deprivation that Rachel suffered when Mark left.

It was my inclination to be very trusting, or maybe the word is even "accepting," of psychological reasoning. But something about Rachel's therapist was rubbing me very wrong by then. I realized that it was not altogether his fault, but I did feel that he, *because* of his training, should have known better than to permit the relationship with Paul to disintegrate. Both were unyielding in their convictions: Ulcerative colitis was not a psychogenic disease as far as Paul was concerned, and he would not be influenced by Klein's advice on his management. In return, Klein regarded the illness almost totally as a psychically triggered problem. Rachel stood between them. Fortunately, it made her more angry than anxious. That day, watching Dr. Klein's smile because he felt that Rachel was fooling us about her eating habits, I suddenly knew that this therapy was doomed as well.

Outside, Mark asked, "How long has Rachel been seeing him?"

"I don't know exactly. Must be close to a year."

"Well, shouldn't he know her better, then? Shouldn't he know that she isn't a cheat?"

"I'd say so!" I had to laugh. No, Rachel certainly was no cheat. She was a fighter; she'd convince us that she *needed* to eat a piece of cake in order to lose weight rather than sneak it behind our backs. I explained my laugh to Mark. "Yeah," he agreed. "And she'd make us believe that the calories of the cake were required to burn up the energy of the coffee she drank."

"Or something."

"A fact about her which Klein doesn't seem to have grasped."

I shook my head. If Rachel ever found out that her psychiatrist didn't trust her, he would be mud.

In the meantime though, the weight came off. Slowly, slowly. Perhaps aided also by the fact that the ulcerative colitis was jiggling her up and down constantly. Home a lot, ill a great deal; she stayed on the harsh regimen.

When the astronauts took the first steps on the moon, she mused, Who knows—now that everything is possible, maybe they'll bring back some substance that can be made into a cure for ulcerative colitis?

By fall 1969 and entry into the new school, she was better and an absolute stunner. With a heart-shaped face, giant golden eyes, and a head of close-cropped curls. Whether she liked the school uniform or not, it became her. And suddenly she was also a tall girl; Paul's management had kept her growing in spite of the disease. In addition to the 6-mercaptopurine and instead of taking the steroids orally, she was now being treated by regular injections of ACTH (adrenocorticotrophic hormone) to stimulate her adrenal glands to produce more of their own steroids. So far, so good. She enjoyed the new school.

APRIL 22, 1977

The fevers have stopped. No one has found an explanation for them. Dr. Gaon, on being pressed, has presented a somewhat simplistic explanation. He says perhaps the high temperatures have literally burned up the infection. Or it has just run its course. I don't know, but I do appreciate his steadfast refusal to go along with rasher suggestions. Once I heard him say to one of his colleagues, "Open her up? Where?" And "Yes, an infection somewhere. No, I don't know where." Enough! Not so some of the others. I am not speaking of the neurologists or the infectious-disease specialists—they were called in as consultants and did not try for much human contact. Some were nice, some almost absurdly impersonal. And each came double. A strange face poking in: "I'm Dr. Whatshisname, Dr. Soandso's associate." Which means that Soandso is playing golf today. Well, never mind them; thank God they have not come up with any awful diseases. That's all I wanted from them.

It's subtly different with the young internist who's been on the case because Paul isn't connected with Mt. Sinai anymore. He came highly recommended by Paul and by Mark's knowledge of him through the Foundation. Handsome too, with a moustache and a lovely bedside manner. He sits on the bed and leans with his right arm on the other side of the body of the patient, therewith making a tent of himself, giving the feeling to the person in bed that his attention is literally surrounding her or him. It may only be for the usual three minutes, but it is effective. However, he also comes in duplicates—there are three of him, in fact. The others are also good-looking and healthy and friendly. Rachel likes all three; I don't. I detect a note of impatience, of insincerity; I overheard a nurse being ordered to retake Rachel's temperature when the fevers were so high. "I want you to stay with her and watch while the thermometer is in her mouth."

I felt myself blushing in indignation, in shame for eavesdropping. I think also in shame for him—to have learned so little about a patient after watching her through this whole ordeal! I guess what I really perceived was his poverty as a human being. An ugly way to react to being stumped: the patient must be at fault.

Yet it makes me think. It's not the first time Rachel has gotten herself disbelieved. Right back to Dr. Klein and the eating. It's a complex, hidden thing, that seems to go unrecognized even by psychiatrists. I call it the "oyster mechanism" in Rachel. She meets new doctors very openly, very cooperatively, in a very friendly manner, and of course, very intelligently. But let her radar pick up distrust or hostility, and she snaps shut. Then she still appears open, cooperative, pleasant . . . only she has stopped giving an inch. She'll sit smiling and answer questions—just what they ask, no more! "Did you tell Robin [as in Batman and Robin; the third associate doesn't have a nickname in our lexicon] about the headache?" I ask.

"No."

"Why not?"

"He didn't ask."

A very familiar pattern of behavior, used on me too when Rachel is angry. I am not sure whether she does it consciously; I think maybe not. And I am almost certain that she does not take responsibility for the tremendous anger which lies behind it. Why, then? Is it a self-destructive tendency? Because certainly she stands to suffer by a mistake or the omission of the right move on the part of the doctors. I think not. I think here is where the tip of the iceberg of her fury shows. Here, consciously or not, she is screaming at "them" (the doctors and us) that they are ignorant and impotent, that they could not save her colon for her. Here she swings the scythe and mows us down, penises and heads flying in all directions; so much hate, so much blood, so much pain.

❦ ❦ ❦

After an x-ray series in November 1969, Rachel wept. It had been even worse than she had anticipated; it had hurt terribly. "The air," she sobbed. "When he pumped in the air . . ."

I drove doggedly, my teeth clenching so that they hurt when I opened my mouth to spout inanities—that it was all over now, all over, that she wouldn't have to go through it again for a whole year.

After a while she calmed down, we were silent. Past Grant's Tomb, she said, "And yet I think that I have had the ulcerative colitis as long as Sam had it, but I don't need the surgery. That's the steroids and the immunosuppressives. And Paul."

"That's right," I agreed.

"I'll bet I'll never have to have it." High after the low.

"I hope not."

"Paul doesn't think I will."

"Did he say that?"

"It's clear. If he weren't sure, he wouldn't make me go through all this junk—I mean, like this morning. And the drugs. ACTH and six-MP. And if he weren't succeeding, I wouldn't have grown."

"True," I agreed again, glad at her mood swing. "And your sexual development would be retarded."

She giggled, looked down her front, and said, "Some sexual development! And I don't have my period yet."

"Patience, Jackass," I quoted from Sam's favorite joke. It was an endless story about an Arab in the desert. He keeps urging his donkey to be patient as they search for an oasis. Sam had a way of dragging it out forever until his listener would say, "So? What happened already?" At which he would shout triumphantly, "Patience, Jackass!"

Rachel laughed on cue, but insisted that just the same, Lonnie already menstruated and she was younger than Rachel. "And Emily, and lots of girls."

"I didn't get mine until I was fourteen. These things are genetic."

Back in New Jersey, on sudden impulse I said, "Let's buy cheeseburgers and sit in a movie."

"I can't. Too much work."

"Okay." I was aching to give her a treat, to make up for the awful morning, but she, apparently, had to compensate in her own manner. By being good and smart and strong.

That night Mark and I sat in the kitchen until very late. Our discussion had started as a result of his angry empathy with the pain Rachel had suffered during the examination. "Was that really necessary?" he had shouted.

I looked at him, surprised. He too? "Come on," I said.

But his face was closed, his eyes avoided mine. "No, I mean it," he insisted.

Suddenly I was beside myself. Another child to deal with. "Do you know of another way in which Paul could make sure that no malignancy is developing than by taking x-rays and a biopsy?" I asked harshly. And when Mark's face contracted as if slapped, I couldn't stop. "Or a surefire test that her colon isn't swelling until it looks like a frankfurter, which, I hear, is how a megacolon looks. A frankfurter that has walls so thin that the likelihood of perforation is ninety to ten . . ." Appalled, I stopped. I had invented the percentage rate; I had no idea what it actually was. What was I doing, why hit Mark?

He had risen and was looking out at the very dark night. Then, turning, he said, "I'm sorry." His voice was tired. He added formally, "I am really very sorry. You know, sometimes I manage to forget."

CHAPTER 7

RACHEL AT SIXTEEN
ON GUSTL'S DEATH:

My mother told me not to be morbid, that there would be plenty of times when I'd be required to go to a funeral, that she was just sparing me. I felt very hurt; she was putting me down; I wasn't important or old enough to grieve for him.

Mark liked to tell the story of how he had wanted nothing so much as to climb into one of those berths in the catacombs beneath Rome. "Lie there and die," he would say, and grin. It made a good tale, how he had exhibited Rome before my eyes with a temperature of a hundred and three which he kept masking from me with aspirin. The reason for this madness was that it was my first time in Rome and our first vacation together during a slot of time when Rachel was well enough to be left. I had discovered the deception at last when, crawling into Mark's bed, I'd found him burning up. It was part of his story now how he told me that it was I who was making him so hot, but that I hadn't bought that theory, had miraculously obtained an American thermometer, and how we had flown home the next day to a seven-week stint of pneumonia.

Sitting in the hot, bright sun at the Ocean Club in Nassau, strummed music in the background, in front of us the aqua sea laced in creamy foam shimmering fantastically, and all the people with us laughing at Mark's story or because they were full of Bloody Marys, I felt a sudden depression so real that it was as if an animal had clawed itself into my chest. Very funny! Seven weeks of pneumonia and the constant up and down of Rachel's condition and Gustl's death.

I thought back: how long ago had it been? In '62 or early '63? The time Gustl had pointed out Paul's article on ulcerative colitis to us? How angry he got because we wanted to read every word. Because he wanted to shield us, because he loved us, had cared. And now he was gone; our world was getting damn low on fathers, while our need of them hadn't abated. And here it was the last day of the year, and what would 1970 bring?

Taking another swig of my drink, I tried to approximate the mood of the others; tried, as if physically, to push off the gloom. Look at all the goodies—a slim Rachel over there in her yellow two-piece suit falling off the water skis, and Sam, skinny, funny Sam, acting disdainful and as if he didn't notice the gorgeous little redhead at his heels. "And everywhere that Samson went, the lamb was sure to go!" Courtesy of one of the besotted adults; the girl's name was Sylvia Lamb, poor lamb. And two of my stories published. And, and—so why couldn't I enter into all the hilarity around me? It was a vacation and everything was okay.

That's what Mark asked me when we were alone in our room. The kids had taken the glass-bottomed excursion boat to see some coral reefs, and our friends decided to see whether their luck would run better in the afternoon in the dark casino. So we had this precious hour alone, and I was moping. I answered Mark that it was nothing. "I'm just so tired. A reaction, I guess. You know, once you let go . . .".

"Courageous by land, courageous by sea," Mark quoted, trying to tease me. It was from a poem Rachel had written about me on the occasion of my last birthday in which things rhymed at the price of credibility.

I gave Mark a sour smile, then said, "Wait, I'll show you," and went through the connecting door into Rachel's room, where I took one of Paul's prescription blanks from her desk and brought it to Mark. "That's what's gotten to me," I said.

In Paul's doctor handwriting it said:

12/23 60 units 1½ cc
27 60 units 1½ cc
31 60 units 1½ cc
1/4 60 units 1½ cc

Mark stared at it, then looked at me. "Her ACTH?" he asked.

"Yes."

"So?"

"So she gives herself the injections now."

He turned pale, and I, now that I was sharing it, became reassuring. "It's okay; she does it very well. Probably a lot better than some strange nurse." We had had our experiences with nurses in hotels.

"But . . ."

And suddenly I was in tears, sobbing and saying brokenly that it didn't make sense to be so upset, to mind, to . . . and tried again: "I mean, why should this seem so horrible?" But the sights of this morning were still before my eyes—a very businesslike Rachel with her cotton swab and alcohol, squinting to read the numbers on the syringe and squirting off an excess cc, explaining to me how it was important not to have any air in the hypodermic, and then plunging the needle into her buttock. The twist of the body to reach herself in back, a dancer's move, graceful, one of the serpents in the last act of *Faust*. "I don't know why it got me so!" I buried my face into Mark's chest.

Which is why I was a wet rag in Nassau. But then slowly, the sun did its miraculous work. Burning itself into the small of my back where the muscles were knotted into a ball of red and black telephone wires, untangling them until the spot felt smooth and caressed, until the wires sang. Then I'd swim leisurely in the incredible waters and suddenly, after some days, I liked my image in the mirror and wanted to go to the casino and to dance and to eat those heavenly meals at La Martinique. And Rachel flew on water skis.

As time went by and the 6-mercaptopurine seemed to hold things together, the thought of the surgery receded. Though I realized that this was odd because, in fact, it had not been consciously in the forefront of our minds—so that it was the *absence* of the expectation of disaster which brought it into the open. At the same time there was the taboo against thinking of the surgery as a disaster because of Sam. And indeed, look at him! And at her, her ups and downs; even at best, never being able to count on her health from day to day. Though we didn't talk about that either. I knew that it was the very precariousness of her situation which made it essential for Rachel to live the "good" days hard, filled and overloaded, stuffed with activities, days she could not bear to end. Going to sleep became harder; Rachel put all of us to bed, then read. I tried to tell myself that it was her rhythm, that she was a night person, that she needed less sleep, but I was not convinced.

Still, we were beginning to understand that the response to the 6-MP was not as dramatic as had been the almost miraculous improvement which the high steroids used to produce during serious exacerbations. No immediate cessation of blood, no sudden end to the pain. But as a supplementary agent to the steroids it was helpful. We also noticed that it was easier and quicker to come off high steroids when they were combined with 6-MP, and the frequency and severity of exacerbation seemed less after Rachel started on it.

"All in all," she explained to a friend on the telephone, "I need fewer steroids now." Walking by, hearing her, I nodded yes, and thought that it also had a good psychological effect on her—she expected it to make her better. She expected to go to school every day, to be finished with her invalid life. And while there were times when she was sick as a dog, she now refused to buckle down to them at all. There were mornings when she had to shuttle back and forth between the toilet and her bed, but by ten or eleven o'clock she'd say that it was better and could I drive her to school. That way she never missed more than a couple of morning hours, and of course, it improved her life; she was a part of the group. Next thing she knew, a boy had walked her home, she had her period, and she played No. 2 on the tennis team. And was "almost fourteen" when asked.

Mark took Sam along to Europe on a business trip that June. Sam was seventeen, five feet ten, and for the occasion had consented to the purchase of a blue suit, clad in which he accompanied Mark to several important meetings with customers. In Germany he served as Mark's translator, using his horrible school German with more cheek than accuracy, and in Italy he stood on the famous steps proclaiming, *"Senatus populusque Romanus!"* The snapshots brought home showed him wearing a navy blue Italian shirt displaying goodly amounts of chest; he and Mark were having a special time. And the trip was just as exciting for Mark as it was for Sam. Spending that kind of time together, taking Sam into his other world—perhaps showing off to the young bull that the old bull was pretty impressive in his own milieu, beyond just being Daddy. Of course, they had always been close, but because of all the illnesses in the house, much of the loving and caring was tied in with being sick, so in recent years Sam had needed to take this love of ours in small spoonfuls. But there in Europe on alien ground, the two were coming together, being friends and men, and, as Mark told it when he came back, he had never even *thought* of asking Sam whether he was all right. "I forgot all the old worries."

Perhaps that seems absurd to an outsider; after all, Sam was then four years postsurgical. But because of the overlapping of the children's illnesses, we had never gotten out of the habit of the watchful eye on them. A friend of ours once accused us angrily of being obsessed with sickness. "God Almighty," he shouted, "Sam's got a simple cold!"

He was right, of course, but he was also completely wrong. Because there was no such thing as a simple cold in our house. To begin with, if Sam had a cold, he was furious. He was furious because, without particularly taking responsibility for the logic, Sam actually felt that he had borne his share of illness and that any more was an insult. I'd try to laugh him out of it and say, "Listen Superman, everyone else gets a runny nose; what makes you so exalted that you're beyond it?" and he'd respond appropriately, but all this did was to drive Sam's anger underground. He'd still be banging doors, throwing Kleenex around, barking hoarsely, and, some six hours after a cold had broken forth in full glory, would begin saying, "It's better already."

Then there was the problem of contagion that made any slight indisposition a problem. Rachel caught everything. Her immune response was definitely impaired by the 6-MP, and a cold in the house was bound to settle in her. Which in turn might, and most often did, start up an exacerbation of the ulcerative colitis. And more anger from Sam: "Why does she have to suffer when she could be well? Why are you so opposed to surgery for her? Look at me!"

It was a dialogue that we had regularly over the years, a conversation in which Mark and I were handicapped by having to be dishonest, or at least, evasive, which was not our usual way with the kids. Because what were we to answer Sam without also saying to him that his ileostomy was not all that desirable to have even if, thanks to his marvelous adjustment and his physical prowess, he had reduced it to a mere inconvenience in his life? And how were we to explain to him that his wish for Rachel to have the surgery as well was not altogether altruistic? Sam, at that period in his development, was aggressively unanalytical, a tendency we felt we had to respect. When I worried that Sam was sweeping every unpleasantness under the rug, Mark used to say that Sam would face it when he was ready.

All of which combined to make a "simple cold" a nonsensical term in our lives, and this was why that trip to Europe at just that time was so important for father and son. It was there that Sam ceased to be Mark's little boy who had been sick. When they came back, the change in their relationship was obvious. And Rachel immediately wanted some of it.

Rachel wanted some of everything now. No, in fact, she wanted a lot of everything. Tennis in the summer was not a set or two, it was six or eight hours of solid playing. And a paper for school was not filling a requirement any old way, it was a serious project into which she threw herself completely. And, as anticipated, she was pushing to leave Dr. Klein because, she said, the sessions were a waste of time and money.

In spite of my own feelings about him, I was not sure that she was right. After all, it couldn't be denied that she had switched into a new gear during the time she had been with him. She had learned to manage herself, the illness, the priorities of her life . . . "Don't you think that all the changes for the better during the last year have had something to do with Dr. Klein?" I asked.

She said no. She said she was simply getting older.

I argued that it took a lot of courage to live her kind of life and perhaps Dr. Klein was teaching her to have the self-confidence that gave her strength.

"Oh, Mom," she said impatiently. "You and your romantic notions about psychiatry!" Then, more angrily: "On the contrary, Dr. Klein kills my confidence. He makes me feel so goddamn guilty with his insistence that I give myself the attacks."

"I'm sure he never said anything of the kind."

"Not directly. But if the exacerbations of the ulcerative colitis are psychosomatic, it follows that something in me wants to be ill. Which puts it all on me."

"That's ridiculous, of course." Now I was angry as well.

"I think so too." Suddenly Rachel was crying. "I have enough to cope with without him."

I wanted to put my arms around her, wanted to say hush, hush, don't cry, sure you can quit. But I didn't. Because I felt that very possibly what she was allowing me to see was just the top layer of a deeper conflict from which she was trying to escape. So I said instead that I wanted her to try it a little longer. "But work on it, discuss these things with him; they belong in his office, not here."

Roughly, she freed herself from my arms, said, "Yeah, yeah, the same old junk! If only you knew what shit it is."

However, and inevitably, the day came when we had to give in and let Rachel terminate the therapy with Dr. Klein. It was done amiably, with the understanding that she could go back if she felt the need. Nice handshakes, good luck, let's be friends, all that.

That evening she came into our bed. She thanked us for letting her quit and said that she promised that someday she'd go and work it all out. "But not now. And not with him." When she left, Mark and I had become convinced that she had made a wise decision.

APRIL 24, 1977

Again and again, as I write this account, I come up against an inner need to explain about having given Rachel so much autonomy so early. Today, the day she is to leave the hospital, it is again obvious that others too are being persuaded by her. I think Dr. Gaon is letting her go a few days before he is absolutely comfortable about her readiness. He's worked out a schedule with her, and she seems to have convinced him that she's capable of doing for herself at home whatever would be done for her here at the hospital.

It's always been that way. Take, for example, the fact that during this last year her professors at college have permitted her to stay registered and that they have agreed to give her "incompletes," which she will make up over the summer. But most often the conflict was with us, at home. Us, me, who have let her make decisions. Sometimes I think of it as a virtue on my part—that I could let go, not clutch. At other times I regard it as a weakness— not being able to stand up against Rachel's steamroller ways, not being able to tolerate her anger at me. But as I look at her now— the way she packs her things; rolls up the posters; stops in between to answer the phone, to chat, to laugh, to already be back in the world—I cannot think of a single decision that I have let her make which I regret. Sure, at each moment of doubt it was always I who'd opt for caution and always Rachel who took the road of peril—the trip to Germany, the half a year in Israel, the university known to be one of the most difficult, the greater course load. Doing everything in spite of the disease. And finally the decision to have the surgery. Yes, the more hazardous procedure.

I feel very strange as I prepare to take her home today. After four hospitalizations, the final time, I think; in a couple of weeks she'll go back to Brown University, to Providence, back into her own life. Not that she didn't bring it along to the hospital too—the books, the paper she wrote for reli-stu (which is not delicatessen but religious studies) on the origin of ethics; the point she makes in it is that ethics need not necessarily stem from religion.

And then there were her mail and her telephone calls and her visitors. She has such very good friends. Starting with Jack, who read her the Megillah the night before the surgery; and all the young people who actually came traipsing down from Providence to sit and literally hold her hand for a few hours. These kids all touch a lot. At first I'd be embarrassed to come in and see some boy sit perched on the edge of her bed, holding her hand, but I have gotten used to it. Now, if some doctor or nurse asks me whether that is her boyfriend, I say no, just a good friend, and I already think them odd for their assumptions. Don't all people touch in friendship? Her girlfriends, incidentally, are physical too. It was especially moving early on when Rachel was still connected to all the tubes and wires. Her friends got in the way, got tangled, but always they wanted to be close, physically close. Nice.

Even the friendships made here in the hospital with the other pouch patients have this intimacy. The day before Rachel's surgery, one of the young women, who was a week postsurgical then, took that first step of courage that's called "getting off the floor" in hospital lingo. With all her bottles and bags and tubes attached, she got into the elevator and came to the seventh floor to wish Rachel luck, to show Rachel that it wasn't long until one rejoined the living. It was horribly moving; we all cried. And it scared me more than it reassured me, because she didn't look so terrific, but for Rachel the girl's act was a great gift.

There have also been visits from other ex-patients. Yesterday Helen came. Looking pretty, cheerful, having come into New York for her two-week-posthospital checkup with Dr. Gaon. The first thing she said was that Gaon told her she could start driving her car—the noble charger spelling independence. Then, up went her skirt. "Look!" Under bikini panties, a small gauze pad over the stoma. And the scar a fine red line up her belly.

"That's all?" Rachel asked.

"That's all."

Both of them beaming. When they started to discuss how soon Helen could have sex, I left. Though they weren't minding me one bit. The course of Helen's illness had been drastically different from Rachel's. She had never known that she had ulcerative colitis until she was pregnant. Then had lost her baby in a violent exacerbation which had also led to immediate surgery. That had been last year. This year she had come in to the hospital for her conversion from the ordinary ileostomy to the continent one which they had not been able to establish under the emergency conditions of that terrible attack. She and her husband were eagerly awaiting the go-ahead for another try at a child.

Altogether, the conversation about babies is most important, coming up again and again among these young women. To everyone's joy, there had already been one successful birth by a pouch patient. Talk of sex is also prevalent, and obviously, a major anxiety, the question of being attractive. Though to me it seems that much of that anxiety must stem from the history of lengthy illness most of them have suffered, the long bouts of fear of incontinence, the feeling about their ugly (bad) bodies which had given them so much pain and which, indeed, had turned ugly on them under the administration of the steroid drugs.

Sitting in the blue chair with my pad and pen in my lap while Rachel is again on the telephone, I dream and think more than I write. I think about the fact that Rachel hasn't had a "boyfriend" since last year, that her one love had shattered on the rocks of the approaching crisis. Not so much, I gathered, a physical problem as that the boy couldn't handle her suffering, the decisions she had to make, the support he might have been required to give. Sensing this, Rachel had walked away. She hasn't talked about it much, and I try to keep my mouth shut, but God, I wish her a wonderful love. Soon, to wipe away all the pain, all the sorrow.

And yet, as I think about it, I know that the young women I have observed here at the hospital in these weeks, while anxious about sex, did not suffer half the fears the boys had. I remember back to the first years after Sam's surgery when I had accompanied him on several visits to other boys who were about to have the same operation. Each time, Paul had called and asked whether Sam would mind speaking to the boy, and Sam had always complied. And while Sam was with the young patient to show and tell, perhaps also with a father in attendance, I was outside trying to make conversation with a mother in horrible distress, a mother for whom I'd feel great empathy, whom I would try to reassure as best I could—look, look at Sam, obviously a shining example of success! Inevitably the question of sex would come up. Would her son be all right? And I would say all the things Paul had pounded into us when we were suffering through that time, about the skill and the experience of the surgeon, about the statistics of success.

Suddenly, as I am thinking of it, I find myself smiling at something I remember. Just before Sam had his surgery Paul had also sent in an ex-patient to speak to him. To Paul that boy had been a triumph—he had grown six inches in the year since his colon was removed; he had been snatched from the doors of death. To us, however, he was a rather small, scrawny, and pimply seventeen-year-old, not exactly inspiring. Nevertheless, Mark, in his extreme anxiety, had taken him aside and had actually asked him about his sex life. To which the boy had replied not to worry, not to worry, he was all right, he was fine. Without exactly saying so, he had given the impression that he was knocking off a couple each Monday and Thursday. Hungry as we were for reassurance, we had accepted this gratefully. Of course, we had not discussed it with Sam—he was only twelve; we had hoped that he wasn't even aware of the possibility of a danger. But some years later, Sam had said to Mark, "Look Dad, I know you have been worrying. So I just want you to know that I'm okay."

Mark had repeated that conversation to me on a stormy November day as we were walking at the beach. Spray was flying, the waves pounded, the wind howled: a moment of some majesty. Suddenly I felt taller, lighter, a burden I had not even consciously acknowledged lifted off my shoulders. It is only now, here, that I wonder, how did Sam know that we were worried? Perhaps because of his own anxiety?

"Hey, Mom!" Rachel interrupts; she's off the phone.

I look up.

"Are you writing nice things about me?" She looks ingenuous; she smiles.

It sends a dart into me, crystallizing an unease that has been growing and growing. Will she, who has persuaded me to write this book—will she like Rachel? I say stiffly, "I'm writing you as I see you."

She laughs. "That sounds bad."

I try for a lighter tone as well; this is not the moment for a deep conversation. I say, "Well, not *too* bad; after all, I'll need you to give me a release if this thing is to be published."

"I want to be a heroine," she says in a high little-girl voice.

And I cannot keep up the banter, feel my eyes fill up, my voice shake. I answer, "You are, Rachel, you are!" But with that the tension bursts like a bubble inside me, and I can suddenly see that this is rather comical—the two of us in the almost stripped hospital room arguing about the image of Rachel in the book. I laugh and promise, "You'll be a heroine, all right; I'll make you your own true self, rotten. Rotten sells books."

But then I see that she is serious after all. Beneath playing at being ridiculous, she is in earnest as she says, still in the silly voice, "I want to be a *nice* heroine."

❦ ❦ ❦

The year 1970 was exciting. For the first time in my life, I was wearing a bikini, because I was going to be a grandmother. And we bought two acres of lovely land in Quogue. It was by a pond and within view of the ocean. I wanted to start building immediately, but Mark had his eye on the two adjoining acres with a marvelous house on them, which he felt must come on to the market soon. So that summer we lived in a rented house again. Only this time, looking across the pond, we could see *our* land. What had gone into the decision to buy was the obvious fact that the kids loved the place as well as we. Both were committed to tennis, to the outdoors, to the kind of relaxed summer living they had known all their lives. Any talk of future plans—working on a kibbutz, getting a job at a hospital—always included a couple of weeks at the shore before or after working.

This summer was a time for serious tennis. Sam's friend Mike, long since dubbed "Coach," worked with him and another youngster again. An attempt by Rachel to be included failed; it was a very macho trio. She retaliated with a furious tennis game of her own, getting to be so good that she was practically snapping at Sam's heels. She never caught up, of course—he was beginning to have weight and speed; but she was good enough to have people saying, "Well, sure, he's older and a boy, but she's really a more natural player."

There did not seem to be any logical explanation for the phenomenon, but ulcerative colitis tended to be somewhat improved during the summer and winter months. With or without understanding why, those of us in the know would say quite matter-of-factly, "Oh, yes, it's spring" when an exacerbation hit. For Rachel too, the summer and winter months were usually the best, as long as she took her various medications, including the daily seventy-five milligrams of 6-MP and the shots of eighty units of ACTH which she gave herself every third week. Which is perhaps why each period of relative calm seduced me into a quasi belief that this was it—the remission. The spontaneous remission—or, okay, the drug-induced remission. Or the one I heard of: "And this girl was practically on the table for the surgery, and then, right after puberty, she was suddenly well!" I'd think cynical thoughts—oh, yeah, for how long? But the tales worked on me just the same, so that each time there was another attack, I'd be completely devastated again.

In September, when Davey was born and we went to Boston for the Bris—the ritual circumcision ceremony—Rachel was in a full-blown exacerbation. I don't know which worried me more, that she'd be able to stay to attend the festivities without flying visits to the toilet or that the *moyel* would clip our little boy properly.

Those were bad weeks. I recall wanting to go back to Boston to get better acquainted with the baby, but was tied to home and chauffeuring Rachel, who was not continent enough to dare venturing out alone. Davey was already five weeks old before I stole a day with him. Feeding him his bottle, holding his smallness, I felt suddenly angry, cheated. Yes, furious that I could not really enjoy this time, be a granny—everyone said it was the greatest! But for me there was only guilt. On one hand because I knew that I wouldn't be with this little boy enough to really get to know him, and on the other hand because I had no business being away from home; it was hard enough for Rachel to manage *with* my assistance. And as I sat there with Davey in my lap, it seemed to me that I'd been a mother forever!

Suddenly I wanted out—and not to be a grandmother, either—out to be me. Finish my book. To write in other ways and places than on scraps of paper, on envelopes, on the back of shopping lists while driving car pools, while waiting in front of doctors' offices, Hebrew school, tennis courts. I thought of a recent time when I'd picked up Rachel at a court. She had been very quiet after getting into the car, and I'd asked her what was biting her. In a tough voice she had answered that it was really nothing, only she hadn't done much playing, she'd been off in the woods most of the time. "I guess they're not about to ask me to make a fourth again," she said, motioning backward with her head toward the kids we'd left behind. "I told them that I had a sudden irresistible urge to commune with nature." She laughed harshly.

Shocked, I kept quiet. Picturing the "woods": a few blocks not yet swallowed by suburban growth, hardly a sheltering forest. And Rachel in pain and mortification. And the kids, thinking what?

I put Davey across my shoulder; I burped him; rebellion trickled out of me like sand out of a torn bag marked CEMENT. Time, I said to myself: time. It was my mantra.

We went back to Nassau for the winter vacation. Suddenly Rachel and Sam looked ridiculously alike: they both wore Afros and were skinny. When they were mistaken for twins, they decided that it was intolerable; Rachel said she'd grow her hair, while Sam would cut his short. Aside from this momentous decision, Nassau was the scene of the fateful walk during which Mark gave Sam the "options speech."

Sam was a junior now. His grades had been consistently good. But not tops. Mark and I, properly brainwashed by all we had read, knew that it was a most heinous crime to put pressure on young people; consequently, we had made no overt comment. On that walk, however, Mark discussed Sam's future with him, asked what college he was planning to attend and whether he was still intending to go to law school. Sam said yes, sure, and he'd sort of like to go to Yale, but he guessed his grades weren't quite good enough. "Though perhaps my tennis will help. . . ."

As Mark told it, his attitude was roughly reminiscent of the one he had exhibited that time when he had been interviewed by the admissions director at Riverdale. I had been present and dying small deaths when Sam, on being asked what he did in his free time, had not discussed his stamps or talked of his trains or even said that he was reading books, but had shrugged and drawled, "Oh, I fool around."

Walking along that dusty road in Nassau, Sam had kicked at

pebbles, had plucked a hibiscus, had whistled. Mark then suggested quietly, "Well, why don't you give yourself some options?" And followed that by a small philosophical discourse in which he had stated that Sam certainly didn't need an Ivy League school to get a fine education, but wouldn't it be nice to have the choice? "I mean, you might decide, as you visit campuses, that you'd prefer the U. of Mo., but, as I said, why not have options?" Sam, grinning broadly, said okay, he got the message.

And indeed he had. He proceeded to settle down during the next year; in fact, by the time he again took that June business trip with Mark (as everything in our life tends to become, it was now a tradition!) he already had a report card of straight A's. His college applications went to pretty exalted places.

Neither Mark nor Sam discussed the U. of Mo. as a possible choice again, though Sam asked me one day whether I thought that this was hurting Mark's feelings. I told him not to be silly. The University of Missouri was Mark's alma mater, where he had been happy and successful; it was also the school that had given him a scholarship, which was the only way he could have gone to college in those days. I refrained from explaining to Sam that this was what it was all about—the Jewish mania for having the kids overtake us.

The result of Sam's new studiousness was a slew of A's and honors, and as I look back, literally look back through the scrapbooks of the next two years, I see that Rachel matched him honor for honor. At Pesach, a special occasion that year because it was Davey's first, we digressed from the Haggadah to discuss the concept of passing on, from generation to generation, the wisdom and lore of the ages. Mark talked of the compulsive status education had in families like ours. Then, looking pointedly at Rachel, he remarked, "Of course, some generations come already equipped with built-in compulsions." To his surprise, the small joke was not well received. The boys defended Rachel ardently. "You should talk," Sam said angrily, and Dan reminded us that the pressure we applied, while subtle, was pretty powerful just the same.

"Yes, from the 'options speech' to 'Why not an A-plus instead?' " Sam added. And, "Not to mention watching *you* work eighteen hours a day."

"I remember when you talked to me about options . . ." Dan began to reminisce, but Ruth interrupted him with the observation that Davey had fallen asleep. Pulling the limp little boy out of the high chair, she said dryly, "Obviously he wasn't feeling pressured yet." It broke up the angry tension that had suddenly built up. But Rachel had the last word. Sighing comically, she said, "And now they have made poor Dan a partner in his law firm. That's what happens to compulsive children."

I listened to them; I looked at them. It was deceptive—the festive table, the candles, the gold-rimmed Pesach dishes, even a baby in a high chair to complete this version of a Seder as painted by some Jewish Norman Rockwell; yes, and even the spice of a kind of anger that underlined our closeness.

The only problem was that it was spring again, a bad time for ulcerative colitis. Rachel had recently commenced daily injections of ACTH; her cheeks were very taut and red and round. I could see that her motor was racing because of the way she took deep breaths; I could hear it in her voice. But there we were. I looked over at Mark in his big white Pesach *yarmulke*, the glasses halfway down his nose, holding the Haggadah: he was listening to the children's comments; he was smiling. And then our glances met and locked, and suddenly I could hardly bear the pain I saw in his eyes. How much longer did we have? Was this going to be the season when Rachel would come to surgery? Because, of course, they always lurked, those perils. The megacolon, the perforation, the malignancy. We could joke and strive for normality and make a pretty good showing of it, but we never forgot those dangers for a moment. I wondered whether Rachel did.

CHAPTER 8

"WHY DOESN'T SOMEONE
DO SOMETHING ABOUT IT?"
"SOMEONE IS . . . WE ARE."

National Foundation
for Ileitis & Colitis, Inc.

On Tuesday, December 14, 1971, it was raining pious words in the Grand Ballroom of the New York Hilton. Twelve hundred people glittered, and the music of Sy Menchen's orchestra pounded. Senator Edmund Muskie had been inoffensive, talking of national-health matters; I had not minded him the way I was minding those who addressed themselves directly to the suffering of the victims of inflammatory bowel diseases. Again and again, "Over one million of them . . ." It was so goddamn much like my six million, *the* Six Million I had evoked myself at all those United Jewish Appeal drives, the way I had sold bonds for Israel, the way in which I had raised money. Okay, so here we were trying to get $200,000 together for research to find the cause and cure.

"We know how it must be done. To find the cause and cure for ileitis and colitis will take time and money for research . . ." from the president of the Foundation. "The progress of the National Foundation for Ileitis and Colitis in its short four growing years has astounded the professionally organized charities across the nation" from his wife, the stalwart Suzanne. Oh, how did she do it? To work so hard, so publicly, with such incredible intelligence, yet be as soft and dear a woman as she was in between her own hospitalizations for ileitis? How many operations had she had? Seven? Something like that, something absurd like that. And here sat I, trying to close my ears, so terribly resentful, feeling that my pain was being exploited with all this hullabaloo.

"We are now in the 'long haul' phase of the Foundation," said the chairman of the National Scientific Advisory Board. "The excitement and novelty of the very existence and formation of our organization has been appreciated by all of us, but now we realize the magnitude of the task ahead . . ." His silly beard! He may try all he can, he still won't look like Freud. Though he is short as well. He was the one we consulted to okay Sam's surgery. The big hand that had affixed the final seal . . .

"Last year's total grant funding . . ." A dramatic pause. Then, loudly, pronounced in separate syllables: "One hun-dred twelve thousand, nine hun-dred and fif-ty dol-lars!" Research at Mt. Sinai Hospital, at the University of Colorado Medical Center, at Johns Hopkins, at the College of Physicians and Surgeons of Columbia University, at New York University Medical Center. Whom was I hating? I was making faces at Nina Zalinger—look at all these awful people, what are we doing here, let's get out! Like a naughty child, I knew. I couldn't stand the rhetoric; I *Couldn't stand it*! Mark shook his head at me. Pipe down, his look said, behave; do you know a better way to raise the money we need? So I subsided, closed my ears. I had a new dress. Long and slim in gray checked wool, a sporty fabric, a sophisticated cut; the dress had a high collar but a naked back. I was cold there. I wanted Mark to put his hand at the base of my neck to warm me; I was freezing.

It's all the pressure, I thought. From absolutely everywhere. Not least of all Rachel's desire to fly to Germany during intersession. She wants to visit Dorothy Bernhard. Dorothy had been our houseguest for three months during the previous fall. The daughter of one of Mark's customers, she had been given the American trip as a graduation present before going to the university. A tall, positive, intelligent, and independent girl—her very posture and striding walk proclaimed an inner freedom—she was a revelation to me, who had only my stereotypes of German children. But for Rachel she was an example. Yes, to travel like Dorothy. "She gets into her Renault and goes to Brussels or Switzerland just like that"—snapping her fingers.

"Dorothy is nineteen, Rachel. Lest you've forgotten, you are only—"

"I know, I know. I am only fifteen and a half. Big deal!"

I refrained from saying that the "half" was also an exaggeration. It was stupid. And now Dorothy's father was sending telexes, friendly letters: "Dear Mr. and Mrs. Bergman, do let Rachel come!" And suddenly we were saying, Well, why not? All right, why not? Hot panic flooding from my stomach outward: What if she has an attack? Among strangers, in Germany yet, hostile Germany . . .

"Don't put your monkey on my back," Rachel had shouted at me that morning. "This isn't the Hitler time, and I don't have your hang-ups."

Sitting in the din of the Grand Ballroom, I thought, Of course, she is right. Truly, I couldn't tell whether my sense of panic at letting Rachel go was realistic. Earlier in the evening, over cocktails, Paul had said causally that he saw no reason why she shouldn't go. "She can always be home in a few hours if there's any trouble." As simple as that. No, it was I. And all this waiting. Waiting for Sam to hear from the colleges, waiting to hear whether Norton would buy the new version of my book. Waiting for the stomachaches I was having habitually to go away. "I can't find a thing," Paul had said after a thorough examination. "You're probably doing too much. Take it a little easier." He had given me a prescription for Librium, which I wasn't taking. I hated the woozy, unfocused feeling they produced. I had to be awake, alert; I had work to do.

I had cut and rewritten my book from page one. True, with some encouragment from the publisher, but without a commitment from that side. Still, I had come a long way—ten stories published, and I had a literary agent. I was also the U.J.A. advisor to the Youth Group that year, the group led by Sam. Such a Sam: calmly authoritative, he had firm leadership. I'd watch him during the meetings, and I'd know him and not know him. The way he handled the kids with ease and charm. And with toughness. A subtle thing—something in Sam was completely unsympathetic to weakness. When a kid complained that he hadn't filled his quota— "Man, they pile it on us in school; I had no time!"—Sam, in a very nice way, told him bull. There is a job to do, we're committed to it, don't give me any sob stories. Nor was he bleeding for the "poor Israelis," either. It was simpler than that: we owe them, Israel is our responsibility as much as theirs, it's the Jewish land; as it is, we don't do much. So he got results, and the kids liked him, but he had distance from them. Also from us. Sam was getting ready to leave home. It would be the kibbutz in the summer and college in the fall; it would be final.

An older woman at the table next to ours dropped her handbag. I bent to pick it up, met her there under the table, saw faded blue eyes and soft wrinkled cheeks wet with tears. "Are you all right?" I whispered.

"Yes, yes, it's just what he said!" The droning speaker. "Our little granddaughter has ulcerative colitis," she whispered back.

I nodded, said, "And our girl too. And one of our boys used to . . ." still under the table.

"Oh, my dear," she said, and squeezed my hand. She sat back again very upright at her table. She was listening to the speaker, paying no attention to the tears that still rolled down her cheeks.

Ashamed, I tuned back in. What was I doing, anyhow? This was my world. I looked at the faces of the men on the dais. They held our fate in their hands; they were good men. They were trying.

I bought Rachel a plastic-lined travel kit for the medication. The tincture-of-opium bottle I wrapped in cotton for extra padding. The hypodermics were in their blue-and-white sterile paper envelopes. I packed a full vial of 6-MP and another to carry in Rachel's handbag in case the luggage got lost. One hundred Prednisone tablets. ("I won't need them!" "Of course you won't!") Cantil, with and without phenobarb, Lomotil, Fiorinal, Librium. "Oh, God, and don't forget to take the ACTH at the last moment!" It had to be refrigerated; she'd give it to the stewardess to keep cold on the plane.

"Mom! *Please.*"

"All right, all right." I burst out laughing. Actually, I wasn't half as nervous as Mark. He had been on a business trip in Germany the previous week; I had a feeling that he had given very explicit instructions to Rachel's hosts. I hoped she wouldn't find out about that.

Then, when her flight was called, hugging her, I held her away from me to study her face for a moment, saw only confidence and excitement, pulled her close once more. Mark, standing behind us, was pale. I signaled to him not to say any more. So we sent her off without a final "Be careful."

Mark did not start the car right away when we got back to the parking lot. We just sat. And suddenly I felt all the knots inside me smooth out, untangle, unravel, be long strands that flowed out of me like colored ribbons around a Maypole; I felt good. "Hey," I said. "Hey—we're alone!" Sam was off skiing. And then we started to laugh. It had been a long time since we had not had any responsiblity; since there had been, literally, nothing we must or could do for our children.

Rachel's first letter was in German; she was able to manage very well. And oh, she loved getting into that little Renault with Dorothy and driving to France for brioche in the morning; she was having an intoxicating taste of freedom, I thought. Her health was not mentioned.

She looked well returning. A tall girl in a navy suit, a girl with elegant legs, golden eyes, and an enchanting smile. She was talking a mile a minute to some fellow travelers when we first spotted her; then greeted me enthusiastically, Mark coolly. And waited until we got home to let go with a barrage of anger at him. Apparently she had found her hosts totally overwhelmed with worry about her health. As the story unraveled, it had taken quite a sharp argument until she had been granted the conventional freedoms. The lady of the house had been prepared to literally wrap her in eiderdown, to feed her a special diet, to insist on ten hours of sleep per night. "Not even Mom has ever been that overprotective! Talk of getting into the fire from the frying pan." In the end, she and Dorothy had taken off, had driven to Munich and stayed with Dorothy's boyfriend, leaving Dorothy's mother worried at home.

Some of the spleen vented, Rachel suddenly turned on Mark and asked, "How could you do that to me, Daddy? You knew how important this trip was."

Mark said that he had simply informed the Bernhards of the nature of the disease; he hadn't asked them to restrict her in this manner; he had been worried.

"But you had no right. What gave you the right?" Tears in her eyes, renewed fury fighting with something else, deeper. I couldn't quite understand what was going on; I interrupted, asked sharply, "What do you mean, right?"

"It's my body, my disease—he's got no right to discuss it with anyone. He's taking away my chance to live a normal life."

"You know he doesn't want to do that; he was worried."

"Tough!" And then an explosion of tears. When she could talk again, she said that it had been hard enough to handle her own fears, her own uncertainties; how could he do that to her, to make it harder, to lay it on her that she was this freak, so ugly, so disgusting?

"Rachel, Rachel . . ." but no stemming the flood; oh, she knew that they were all trying to be nice to her because they felt sorry, but she was trying so hard, ". . . and the trip was so important. I thought, If I get there and no one knows—I knew that Dorothy wouldn't tell, wouldn't make a fuss; she was terrific when she was here too; she sort of ignored the whole business—I thought, If I can handle it there, among strangers . . ."

I began to understand; thought back to her facial expression before leaving: nothing showing; an act of will, of courage. Mark had gotten up, was walking over to where Rachel sat in the low orange armchair. He pulled her up by her hands. She came up reluctantly, but then was in his arms. "I'm sorry, I'm sorry," he kept saying, and finally the stiffness went out of her body and she let herself lean against him. She let herself cry.

Later, with coffee cups in our hands, all of us red-eyed, we really talked. Once the problem of Mrs. Bernhard had been settled, it had been terrific. "But Mom, you have to write to her and apologize—I did, a million times—she was in such a bind. Imagine having a scene, with tears and all, with a visitor. When she meant so well . . ." And all about what she and Dorothy had done, where they had gone, what they had eaten. I kept waiting, but no word about the colitis; nor did I dare ask. However, I did make the other *faux pas*. Looking at my watch: "My God, it's eleven; that's five o'clock for you!" Smiling, Rachel raised a warning finger at me. "Please, Mom! This has to stop." Then seriously, "You'll have to trust me to manage."

Groaning inside, I said okay humbly enough. And in another hour, when my own not-jet-lagged strength had run out and I was in bed, and while Mark was still brushing his teeth, Rachel came and sat with me. She took my hand; she said, "Look, don't get upset, but I'll have to call Paul tomorrow. I'm afraid I have to see him."

The *bête noire* was back on my chest, claws and all. I asked, "When did it start?"

"Four, five days ago, but I knew it was coming."

"How did you manage?"

"I gave myself two extra shots of ACTH, but it didn't help. The last couple of days I took the opium."

I nodded, then had to raise the other thing that was driving me crazy: "Rachel, you said before that you're ugly, a freak. I hope it was in the heat of battle—a few dramatics, huh? You know that you're a beautiful girl—"

"Oh, Mom!" she interrupted impatiently.

"Oh, Mom, nothing. Listen, when we saw you come out of Customs . . . why, you're a stunning-looking girl!"

"Yeah, to you. A Jewish Mother's Heart. No"—she shook her head; she wasn't fooling, she wasn't fishing. She said seriously, "No, I'm pretty disgusting. And wait how I'll look after Paul's hiked up the steroids!"

Tired or not, I couldn't sleep for a long time that night. For the first time, I think, I had a sense of the depth of Rachel's negative feelings about herself—an almost incredible lack of reality judgment in the face of her looks, her success with people, her accomplishments in school and in sports. And again felt a confirmation of my determination to help her be independent. Only on her own could she prove her worth. My reassurances were simply froth, not really pertinent; I was the doting Jewish Mother, at best an unreliable thermometer.

Paul confirmed the bad tidings. Rachel decided not to go back to school after her appointment with him. "First day after vacation, all we do is fool around!" So we had a long afternoon of talk; we watched it get dark in her room. In some weird way, there was always a moment of peace, even luxury, when we first had confirmation of trouble. It was almost a relief, after the anxiety, because it took energy to deny the obvious. Very quickly after that there would come a gathering of forces for the fight back, for the climb up, but for just that one moment it seemed proper to be overwhelmed. That was the spirit of the afternoon.

MAY 2, 1977

When I began to write this account and decided on the technique of going back and forth between the present and the past, the present was centered on Rachel's operation; indeed, I actually started the book that morning while she was in surgery, just as I had promised her. I did only about a page—couldn't concentrate—but it was a gesture of faith, a statement that I believed that a moment would come when that morning of surgery would also be the past, would be wrapped in the fine mist of time, its agony under at least a local anesthetic of perspective. For Rachel, making me promise that I would begin writing *her* book at that moment, it must have signified a tie to survival.

In the meantime, with Rachel home and well on the road to recovery, this section of each chapter that I write in the present has become a sort of diary. Because writing this book has become curiously lonesome as each of its characters withdraws from it and from me in confusion.

To begin with, Mark. After reading a few pages, he said, "I don't know how you can bear to do this." And soon Sam, angry, afraid of the invasion, the cracking of the shell of our private egg. Only Rachel remained interested for a while, but then became uneasy that my perspective would not be hers. So that now this is all mine while they stand back, fastidiously; not really hostile, just reserved. Lonely business.

Today, when I come home from marketing, there are four pouchies around the dining-room table. I knew that Rachel planned to meet the others at Dr. Gaon's at noon; they were going to have lunch in New York after their checkups. But apparently they had all been too tired to fight the crowds, and Rachel had suggested coming here. They all look well, tanned and lively. I join them and we laugh a lot, mostly about the doctors, who all have nicknames—all except Dr. Gaon, who is not even "David" to any of us—and about the nurses like Norma, whom, after all, they are all attached to, who was everyone's link to a return to life. Somehow the very annoyances with which she rubbed made her so important. And Nanette, who has become Rachel's friend. "And the beautiful black girl, what was her name? She spoke so softly." "Altha!" "Yes, Altha!" I also hear, as I listen to them, that I did not know every last thing that went on—as about the doctor who made passes. "Why didn't you tell me?" I ask, amazed.

"It was so damn upsetting at the time; I was still pretty shaky. I just didn't want you to get into it." She adds in a tougher voice, "I handled it."

A wave of sickness rises in me. I had thought him so nice, so gentle; what kind of sick is that, to molest a patient? Yes, molest. But the girls have passed over this already; Rachel was not the only one favored by him. They talk of summer plans. Joan, the one who had come to visit with all her tubes and bottles on the day before Rachel's surgery, will travel to Mexico. "Wow, Spanish food, how I love it." Wow indeed. Is she different from the scared sparrow of that other day! And it turns out that everyone is already eating everything, including the forbidden Chinese vegetables and mushrooms.

Sitting with them, hearing what they say—Rachel is the youngest; the oldest is only thirty-one—I think they sound like a bevy of schoolgirls. Strange, they seem to care enough about their commonality to keep up the contact, to meet as friends. On the other hand, they are very superficial in their touch. Tentative; better to laugh a lot. It's one more thing that Rachel appears to handle differently from Sam. Shortly after his operation, we had gone to an Ostomy Club meeting. But only once; he rejected it angrily. I argued, said that a lot of people obviously found comfort in these meetings; but Sam said no, not he. "What a crazy idea that I'm supposed to have something in common with someone just because we had the same kind of surgery!"

When he is annoyed with Rachel, he'll cite this otherness, point out that she does things that are foreign to him. But not really, I think. Because it's just a matter of style, a surface thing. Yes, she seems more open, less reserved, but you can walk in on her only a short distance. Then there is a locked door. And I, between being afraid that I am being invasive and my various concerns about her, I can only focus on her psychiatrist, Dr. Freund, and hope that he helps her to know herself.

Locked doors are fine if the owner has the key. But Dr. Freund or not, how very, very hard it must be to now acknowledge all the fear and anger and alienation that she kept hidden so successfully during the years in which denial was necessary just to cope. Though this may only be my conjecture because it was *my* way of living with the illness once removed, and perhaps Rachel faced it more realistically than I? Perhaps, inside, she'd been preparing herself for the inevitability of the surgery all along? But no, I shake my head. No, Rachel and Paul had both been absolutely sure that the medical management would work for her; they had been crusaders on a quest. Yes, and with each passing year their investment in that belief had become weightier. Oh, certainly during the last few years Rachel's faith in Paul and in the drugs had solidified into a shield that had protected her even against the worry about chromosome damage in connection with the 6-mercaptopurine and it had kept her awareness of pain at bay. . . .

"Why are you shaking your head?" Rachel is asking. I wake up again to where I am, the sunny dining room, the young women around the table; they are all looking at me.

"I was just thinking," I say, feeling embarrassed, caught at it. "I was thinking how worried we used to be before the operation. Because we never knew how much pain Rachel was in and whether she denied pain by act of will or unconsciously. . . ."

"I bet," Joan agrees. "Pain is a barometer of the condition; it's dangerous not to know how much there is." She turns to Rachel, says mockingly, "Bad girl."

But Rachel laughs. "Ah, you know parents!"

And then they all laugh and so do I. What else?

❦   ❦   ❦

Rachel fancied herself grown up after that trip to Germany. And in fact, I didn't give her much trouble because she acted like an adult most of the time. Though there were a couple of problems: school and Paul. School was beginning to seem irrelevant to her. Why couldn't she plan to graduate after her junior year? Everyone knew that a senior year was a total waste of time.

Mark and I put our collective foot down firmly on that one. "You'll just have to suffer it," I said with little sympathy.

"But even the junior year will be a drag. Look what's a requirement!" She stabbed her finger on the word RELIGION on the schedule that lay on the table.

"What's wrong with religion? I thought it interested you." In fact, she had been getting very active in the synagogue.

"Yes, but not in *school*! Mom, really, under religion they still mean those Gentile gentilities, junk that goes with round-collared young ladies' blouses." The school had barely recovered from its antiuniform crusade; it had also merged with the adjoining boys' school, which I had believed would render it more interesting for Rachel. But apparently not.

"I think I'll ask to do an independent study for religion!" she declared. I groaned; she laughed. She had lost the battle to go to college early, but I knew we had lost the war "not to give her extra pressure," which had been Mark's and my objective in not considering letting her graduate too young. And the words "independent study" were horribly reminiscent of the hematology craze. "I hope you'll pick something with a beginning and an end," I said.

"Very funny." She shook her head judiciously, thinking, planning.

I suppose it was a question of making independent judgments. The school approved her suggestion for an independent study when she presented an outline for looking into "Death and Dying in Today's Society." It was just at a moment before it became a generally accepted topic. Kubler-Ross was probably the only name anyone recognized. Mark and I had no objections. In fact, hearing Rachel pose the questions she proposed to investigate, I was very much interested to hear her conclusions. I only feared that she was embarking on another big trip—she intended to read mythology, Freud, the poets, as well as analyze present-day customs and attitudes.

I don't know whether it was the kind of respect she encountered from her teachers or—the only bonus the illness seemed to provide —a kind of self-confidence, or perhaps experience, that assured her that she could manage in all kinds of difficult situations, but Rachel truly assumed that it ought to be up to her judgment to decide when she was to see Paul as well. She also wanted to have a say on whether or not x-rays were necessary and how much medication to take.

I thought Paul was rather long-suffering in the way he permitted her to share all these decisions with him. But I did not quite understand something he said to us at that time—namely, that it was too bad that Rachel found it so difficult to accept guidance and that he did not think that she could receive optimal medical attention as long as she would not yield some control. Looking back, I realize that I quite misunderstood the statement. I took it to be critical; I thought it unworthy of him to engage in a power struggle with the child, and I remember vaguely defending her. I do recall my angry thoughts clearly: You try it, Paul, you try having ulcerative colitis and see whether control doesn't become an obsession with you too!

Later I found that I was not the only person intimately involved in the management of ulcerative colitis who found it difficult to be balanced on the question of control. At a seminar the Foundation opened to the public, a panel of doctors presented their views, then answered questions. I sat next to a burly fellow who was listening attentively. But when one of the doctors answered a question pertaining to life-style with a rather abstract and hifalu-tin thesis on overcoming obstacles, he jumped to his feet and shouted, "Yeah, try it once with the shit running down your legs!" And I, startled, embarrassed, horrified, found that I felt a wild rise of answering resentment against the speaker on the dais as well as a sense of empathy and understanding for my rude neighbor.

In retrospect, I understood what Paul had meant. It wasn't a question of criticism, more a statement of fact. Right or wrong, understandably or not, Rachel was a difficult patient for him. Of course, there was an incredible amount of ambivalence in her emotions toward him, and it was all complicated by the friendship. For me too—I continued to have stomachaches.

But when we took Sam to his plane to Israel for a summer on a kibbutz, there was a moment when my cup ran over; I didn't have a single worry about him. Paul had checked him, had suggested that he take some extra salt pills and drink a lot, but that he could otherwise do anything he chose; he was a strong, healthy young man; he was going off to do something we all considered of the highest worth. And he had been accepted at Yale. Waving good-bye, he was cocky as all hell.

So was I. My book would be published in February of the next year, and we had bought the other two acres with the house on them.

Paul and Nina spent the Fourth of July weekend with us, and I read them Sam's first letters. He was starting work at four thirty in the morning, he was working in the banana fields and sometimes in the fishponds, the other volunteers with whom he bunked came from Argentina and Switzerland, and he was hitchhiking to visit the Israeli division of our family over Shabbat. He was feeling great; he had met his friend Ben, an Israeli kid who had been an exchange student at Riverdale the previous year; they were planning to do some touring together. Looking up from the letter, embarrassed because there was nothing to cry about in the text and yet the tears were rolling down my cheeks, I found the others moved as well. It was inevitable that—together—we had to think of little Sam with the jutting shoulder blades and the bravery against impossible odds.

Rachel, momentarily out of the center of attention, did fancy dives off the springboard; she was having a good summer too.

But the following winter was bad. All the nice productivity to which she had become accustomed was interrupted by a terrible attack of ulcerative colitis. It took a big bite of time. And toward the end of it, Paul said to me, "You know, I can't leave her on the six-MP forever."

"Why? Are her blood tests bad?" Immediate panic like a wave.

He shook his head. "No. No, as a matter of fact, it's been agreeing incredibly well with her."

"Then why can't you leave her on it?"

"The next time she has an extended period of no activity, I want to take her off." Ignoring my question.

"But there hasn't even been an extended period of no activity *with* the six-MP," I protested.

"Even if she has low activity," he insisted.

"But why?"

Which was when the telephone rang at Paul's elbow. By the time he had hung up, I could not get my courage back to ask that "why" again.

CHAPTER 9

"Well, not to be Pollyanna-ish about it, it was probably the best year and the worst year of my life"

Rachel, May 28, 1977

MAY 28, 1977

We are in Quogue, our first weekend in the sun; Nanette is with us. It is unbelievable . . . I mean, it always is, the three-ring circus nature puts on. Yesterday's weather change, for instance. I watched the whole drama, overwhelmed, as the calm pond—dead still in two-tone gray, the foreground like a Parisian kid glove, in back ominously soft, the gray of doves—began suddenly to stir. First a wind and the waters starting to roil and excited birds flying up and landing in senseless choreography on the choppy waves. And then the mists rolled forward, eating more and more of the pond, and finally the rain, a curtain.

Today, perfect beauty and serenity. And I realize why I see everything as through a magnifying glass—the beloved sights which are, this weekend, outlined in charcoal because we are here. Here, in contrast to being elsewhere. Here, not in the hospital. We are here; Rachel is lying on a towel by the pool; she is tanning her belly; she is wearing a bikini. Of course, this reminds me of a scene a couple of weeks after the surgery when Dr. Gaon was checking her scar. He had nodded, said in a satisfied voice, "Fine; you can wear a bikini this summer."

Rachel had protested: "But I never do. I'm too fat."

"Nonsense. Now you shall."

Obviously Rachel feels that it is a matter of pride, the least she can do for Dr. Gaon, for his beautiful work. But she is shy; when the grocery boy comes, she covers up.

I was up early, before seven. I made myself coffee and came outside to savor waking up and being alone; I was sure that everyone else was sleeping. But then Rachel came walking across the lawn from the direction of the ocean. "You should have seen the sunrise!" she exclaimed. In her hand, a pad and pen. I asked, "Did you record it?"

She laughs, embarrassed. "Don't worry, no competition." Then, "Maybe I'll start writing a journal." She hesitates, then says, "Can I read you what I wrote?"

"Of course, if you want."

But instead, she gives me the pad. "Here, you read it." And adds, hastily, "If there's anything in it you can use for the book, you're welcome to it."

I thank her and watch her go into the house. And then read these pages:

Daybreak in the dunes. The ocean is very meek and the pond glass still. I've just watched the fiery red moon slip away, now the horizon is pink as a soft peach. It's almost light, the day is born, one pastel is fading into another. And the sound of the waves. Most of all, the smell—salty, fresh; sea and sand. I like to be alone and awake and here. My soul craves this peace. If only I sit here long enough, perhaps it will seep into me, maybe it will soothe the hurt of the last years.

It's almost summer now. The last time I came to the beach to watch the sunrise the summer was about to end. But it was so different—then, I hadn't slept all night because the high doses of steroids which I was taking kept me too stimulated. Tonight, returned, I was also awake. Tonight my excitement was of a different sort altogether—I've been trying to really believe that the last twelve years are now a part of my past rather than an ongoing, integral part of the present and future.

It's hard to conceive that all the pain is behind me. Looking back, it seems such a Herculean load to have had to bear. And while the surgery and the past few months of recovery have been no picnic, my chance to live a normal life has been restored. Last year I couldn't have written that line. Last year I was still too busy denying, too busy maintaining that I was living a normal life—with just a few minor exceptions—the whole ordeal nothing more than parenthetical . . . After all, I thought, if I could do that, things couldn't be so bad.

And yet I was in despair when I was here last. Alone, on a deserted beach, no one to pretend to, perhaps I suddenly had the freedom to see, for just a second, that things couldn't go on the way they were. And I cried. And I called out to God—trying to hide my anger—if only he'd help me. Though I did not know what form that help should take. Or did I? They say He works in mysterious ways—well, at the risk of being irreverent, it feels like I did most of the work. And I wonder how long I'm going to feel so devastated, so wounded, so invaded. Or do I want too much, too fast?

Here comes the sun. The sea gulls are making this terrific racket, thinking themselves roosters, yelling rise and shine to the world, not to miss this new and beautiful day. That's the point, isn't it? Each day is new and beautiful for me now. I will just have to believe it, in spite of the ups and downs. What a lot of adjusting I'll have. But when I think of all the repressing and denying I've done over the years—that's something I can only allow myself to see now. And this permission hurts. It's too mild to speak of indignities. It's an understatement to talk of pain. And lost childhood and confusion and isolation. . . .

🌷 🌷 🌷

After a while my vision blurred, I hunted for a Kleenex in my bathrobe pocket, I blew loudly; what had gotten me was the word "indignities." I wanted to read on, but here came Rachel and Nanette, laughing and giggling with their coffee mugs. And Rachel took the pad out of my hand and said, "Gross, isn't it?" And didn't wait for an answer. Nanette has skin as white as snow, never-in-the-sun skin; I ran for the sun-screen lotion—"You'll burn to a crisp if you aren't terribly careful," I warned—and they humored me and Nanette put on the lotion. Then they spread themselves out like slices of lox and waited for the sun to paint them beautiful.

At the very end of 1973 we were enjoying a few days at the new house in Quogue. At last it was free of workmen; we had glorious fires in the hearth and the wonders of the winter ocean's roar, and we walked in the mingled snow and sand at the beach. Both Rachel and Sam had brought work and spent a lot of time in their rooms; Mark and I kept saying over and over again how much better this vacation was than going to Nassau and other points south. Because we were tired; it had been another difficult year.

Early in the spring, within two weeks after taking Rachel off the 6-mercaptopurine, Paul had to put her back on it. It was soon enough to prevent the attack from becoming really bad, so that Rachel was able to limp through the spring. She was too busy to be sick; she was playing on the tennis team; and after handing in the fine paper she had done on Death and Dying, she persuaded the school to let her teach a course on the subject to enrich her awful senior year and because she thought that it would be a good experience for other kids as well. To remove the taboos . . . "Almost everyone has had death in their family," she argued passionately, and said that the kids needed to talk about it. After discussing it with various teachers, a minister, the rabbi, and a psychologist involved with the National Thanatology Society of America, she was encouraged. The school made an inquiry whether there was student interest and netted twelve sign-ups.

Sam, hearing about it, was outraged. "Don't tell me about it," he yelled at her over the telephone. Mocking, scolding, punishing with contempt. "You creep! Don't we have enough?"

What was enough? In May, after Rachel and I had sent out invitations to all our friends to come celebrate Mark's fiftieth birthday with us, my father died and we had a funeral instead of a party. A funeral, and the grotesqueness of the same friends around the open grave. Very unreal on a beautiful hot day. A month later the dog was killed—and at last there were all the tears we had been too shocked to cry before. And then my book had come out and given me escape. Because I was suddenly hit by a terrible urgency to write the next one, drunk on the feeling I would get wandering into bookstores, standing and looking at my book on display, thinking of the reach and the touch—perfect strangers would be connected to me. So I wrote away madly in the midst of carpenters, painters, and electricians in the new house. Not to mention Rachel and her friends. Sam had been home on weekends only; he had worked in a textile mill over the summer. And then in the fall, the Yom Kippur War. Thunder struck into our hearts, and both children wanted to go to Israel immediately.

Yes, enough. We were tired. And the issue of Israel was in no way resolved. Sam would go next summer and lend his hands to the kibbutz again, but Rachel wanted to go for six months. And apparently was winning Paul's support for the idea. She had already persuaded her school to let her take off the last semester, in lieu of a senior project, and she was working on us. "Paul said that he saw no reason for me not to go as long as I don't take on the hardship of kibbutz life. I can live in Jerusalem and learn Hebrew and work in a hospital." And Paul agreed that he would not take her off the 6-mercaptopurine again until after she came back. We were still arguing, but without much expectation of success. I asked, "What about your graduation?"

"Who cares about that?"

Back and forth.

For New Year's Rachel was going to have a boy visiting. Boyfriend? She wasn't sure; she wasn't sure whether she liked him all that much. He was a little peculiar. ". . . you'll see, Mom."

He seemed cute to me, tousled dark hair and very smart, and he loved music. Maybe he talked a little too much, but he handled Sam's humor well. Sam was sometimes a little rough on Rachel's male friends. To begin with, he wasn't crazy about having to share his room, but more than that, he displayed an old-fashioned kind of resentment—an almost "what-are-your-intentions, sir?" kind of attitude. As for Rachel, it was clear to me that indeed she didn't quite know how she felt about him. He made her laugh a lot—a nice new kind of laugh. Mark met my eyes at dinner and pulled up his eyebrows. But then on New Year's Eve, after Mark and I had gone to bed, Mark decided to get up once more to check whether the fire was properly banked. He was back under his covers in a jiffy, somewhat traumatized by the sight of Rachel and the boy kissing by the fire. His little girl! However, it was clear the next day that the kisses couldn't have amounted to much; when the boy declared that he had to join his parents for a traditional January First visit at his grandparents', Rachel seemed almost as relieved as Sam.

I didn't know whether it was the anxiety of this not-quite-ready-for-it-yet romance or the signs of renewed trouble, but Rachel became very much depressed on our last day of vacation. I found her crying in her room. "Do you want to talk?" Sniffling, "No. Yes." I waited. She was so tired, she said. She was so tired and she had so much to do. She had to prepare the paper she had been asked to present in March at a seminar sponsored by the National Thanatology Society which would convene at Presbyterian Hospital; the Society wanted her to discuss her experiences in teaching a class on Death and Dying to high school students. The class, which was a great success, was proving to be very hard on her; predictably, she took it very seriously. The pride and pleasure it gave her to teach it—a local minister and a Ph.D. candidate in theology came regularly to listen in, and the minister had mistaken her for a grown-up teacher—were offset by the responsibility that weighed very heavily.

"It's like lava pouring down once they start," she had said. "Once they know that it's okay to talk of their grandfathers' deaths." And everything had become more complicated because a boy in her school had dropped dead one day. Just walking along the corridor with a bunch of them, he had fallen down and been dead; a boy who had been on the football team. It appeared to Rachel that her class was looking to her for leadership, for inspiration, on how to handle themselves in this terrible situation; the fire was a lot hotter than she had anticipated.

Later, all four of us walked to the beach. In the winter the sun sets into the ocean. That evening it sank quickly, dramatically, flushing the sky red, then pink, then mauve, while the gray clouds had golden borders. Then suddenly it was dark and very cold; we hurried home. Next morning we left the winter paradise—the pines bent under their heavy snow cushions; the steel gray pond from which squadrons of wild ducks took off and landed in formation; the pheasant family that marched across our snowfield, leaving delicately edged footprints like a ribbon of lace in a wedding-dress train. Back to work.

The paper for the Thanatology Society was quite a revelation to Mark and me. Rachel called it "On the Fighting of Preconceived Notions" and basically made the claim that it was the projected anxieties of the adults around her about death that made family deaths the unreal ordeals they were for her. Oh true, true! Rachel's thesis: if adults could only accept, then children could and would if permitted to. And that teaching the class, she had been caught in tangled bands of steel until the resistance had smoothed and the children felt free to talk.

I thought the paper was excellent and her reproach of our attitude justified. Another thing I found interesting in her thesis was her calm assertion that her desire to be a doctor was probably a counterphobic defense against all the sickness she had suffered, all the deaths in the family, and a reaction to her own fears. It was not a surprising thought for me, but I found it startling that Rachel was having so much insight. Again, with mixed feelings, there was a reminder that she was growing up terribly quickly.

And so we sent her off to Israel in April. In her red passport case she carried a letter from Dr. Dash instructing Whom It May Concern to do blood and platelet counts on the above-named patient at three-week intervals. She also had a letter from Dr. Paul Zalinger giving her medical history and another that listed the medications she must carry. A long list, including: "... ACTH gel, which requires two or three cc syringes," lest she be arrested as a drug addict. We kissed good-bye with tears and laughter. She tried to soothe Mark's fear by exclaiming, "Daddy, I'm seventeen!" "Yes," he had answered. "Right." And then she was gone, disappeared into the security area, and a young Israeli guard, no doubt addressing himself to our expressions, said to us, "There is no safer place than an El Al plane!"

But of course it wasn't just the letting her go into a country barely out of war, a place reverberating with terrorist activities. No, our main concerns were other people's trivia—strange water, other foods, diarrheal disorders: what would these normally innocuous disorders do to Rachel? And if she had trouble, would there be a doctor who would know enough about the disease and the drugs Rachel was using to orchestrate proper management, or would she feel that her own judgment would be better than some strange doctor's? We had encouraged her not to hesitate to call Paul, but of course, in any really serious situation she would have to come home. But would there be enough time? And what would it do to her to fail? Because that was the way she would regard it, as a failure. I said out loud, and my voice was rough, "... which is no reason not to let her try it. She can't let fear cripple her." And Mark nodded, completely tuned in on my thoughts. Yes, well, that was why she was on that plane.

Then, still communicating in that extraterritorial region, Mark added, "But we have to live too."

"We'll live," I said. "We'll get used to it."

And indeed we did. Though I felt better once Sam was also there and better still after we had visited in June. And seen her in her aerie, an apartment in the new section of immigrant housing, up many flights of stairs, extremely primitive, but beautiful because everything built of the white Jerusalem stone is beautiful, and lovely with the stamp of Rachel, her laundry fluttering on the clothesline outside her window. We had also seen her go off each morning to her *ulpan*—her language school—and heard how proficient her Hebrew was getting to be. But mostly, we had seen her at her job at Hadassah Hospital. She was working in the Respiratory Intensive Care Unit, operating all kinds of therapeutic machines and assisting in the various procedures. We went there one evening to pick her up. It was seven o'clock, then seven thirty. Outside a green door we waited. When someone came out, we peered in. In those seconds we saw a large room and beds and patients and white-clad figures moving about, and finally we had a glimpse of Rachel bending over a still form. Then the door swung shut.

"Was that Rachel?" Mark asked.

"Yes."

"First I thought it was a doctor."

"Because she's wearing a white coat." My heart was pounding hard. Though I did not know precisely why. How could they let Rachel do such serious work? But I felt pride in her. And fear—so damn much reality. Around eight o'clock she came out. Indeed in a white coat and stethoscope! A boy, a soldier, was very bad, and one of the nurses had become sick; she simply couldn't leave.

On the way back to the hotel I was suddenly aware—oh, and as sensitive as to the screech of chalk on slate, skin-crawlingly sensitive—of the knowledge that all those handsome boys in the streets didn't carry their guns slung over their shoulders for fun. Or to play cowboy games. And Rachel was most familiar with this awareness. At one A.M. that night she cried. It was from exhaustion and because the young soldier would soon be dead.

Still, we left her there. In fact, we left with a modicum of peace of mind. I understood her need to be a part of Israel at just that moment. I think I also understood her need to be on her own. Or perhaps just to be away from us.

And then it was the end of August and both Rachel and Sam were back. We went out to Quogue. Sam looked skinny and green; he had worked very hard. All the sharks at the club were glad; this time they would beat him in the tennis tournament he had won the previous year. But on his first day back after almost losing to a man who was Mark's and my age and had ten children to boot, Sam pulled himself together and started playing. And won once more. Rachel, who had come in second the year before, did not feel like competing at that time. She and I were having a rough time at home; almost everything I said and did was an invasion of her autonomy. I was glad to think that it wouldn't be for long. Rachel had been accepted at Brown University and would start her freshman year in September.

Rachel thought that going away to college would be a snap. She would have none of the freshman separation *Angst*, not after spending six months in Israel by herself. And perhaps that would have been so if she had not gotten sick so quickly after the start of the school year. Installed in a coed dorm, she was given a room-mate vulnerable to infections, and they set off trading colds, flus, earaches, and coughs. Until doctor's orders separated them and Rachel had the luck to be able to remain in the nice large room by herself. But by then it was too late. A serious exacerbation laid her so low that she could barely manage to get herself to classes. It made the work load impossible. The high steroid doses kept her too stimulated to sleep; the painkillers dazed her, made it hard to stay alert; and she had embarked upon a heavy academic program. However, she insisted that it had to be done that way. I later wondered how much of an unconscious realization there had been even then that a time would come during which she would have to carry a lighter course load.

Just the same, and while her grades suffered—which is the great-est catastrophe in the life of a premed—she managed a college life. True, she did not go to parties, smoke pot, or drink. I think that was partly for medical reasons and partly because she had an ab-horrence of self-destructive behavior, and she certainly considered the pot and drug craze to be in that vein. But also, perhaps, be-cause when she had active ulcerative colitis, Rachel not only felt herself threatened by the chance of incontinence, but considered herself unattractive. Strangely enough, this did not really hurt her social life. She found friends who accepted and/or shared her atti-tudes. Some of them were oddballs, all were interesting kids, none were of the very glamorous fast crowd. She also had a disappoint-ment to deal with when a romance that had barely budded at the very end of her Israel stay came to naught at home, where the differences in mores between this very Orthodox boy and Rachel's enlightened views on Judaism loomed larger than when they'd gone backpacking to Elat in the camaraderie of the Israeli life-style.

We visited Freshman Weekend. Rachel's room, with its enor-mous chair from the Salvation Army, its array of blooming plants, its Israeli batiks on the walls, was a bit of home. She also had a cat which smelled awful and which, I think, she wouldn't have minded being rid of if it could have been done honorably. I was worried because she looked very ill, her skin transparent and with deep purple shadows beneath her eyes. But I was also reassured that she had dug out a niche for herself. Kids were in and out of the room—Rosemary on crutches, who told me that Rachel had driven her to the hospital when she had her accident, and Jan, who said that Rachel had practically written his psych paper for him. Obviously she was being who she needed to be again: the helpful one, the one who listened, who fed the others. Her own diet was terrible; she was trying to counteract the steroid weight.

CHAPTER 10

OPEN YOUR HAND

Open your hand, let go.
Give up that gesture you have practiced
                    since before thought . . .
that instinct
to clutch the finger that fits your palm.

Open your hand.
If you let go, it will let you go.
You might soar or lie on a cloud.
Or walk away.

Open your hand.
Wiggle the fingers, free.
Stroke yourself, your nice velvet skin.
Hold a mug of hot coffee.

JUNE 1977

Rachel has gone up to Providence. And I wrote a poem, this poem. The first in all those years. And while I wrote it, I did not know whether it was about Rachel or about myself. Yes, Rachel was scared to go. School is almost over; then all her friends will leave and she will be alone in a strange house working, doing her research. And she is still not allowed many activities. So it was very difficult for her to leave. Go, darling, go, I thought; perhaps, if you're not afraid, you will lie on a cloud. Oh, yes, the poem was about Rachel, for Rachel. And then the last verse flowed out of me . . .

Oh, open your hand and let go.
What can happen even if you fall?
As in the beginning,
*   you are close to the earth . . .*
No longer young.

And I knew it was about me. It is I who want to walk away, I who do not know that I can make it without the fear that has been the ramrod up my back, that has kept me going. And I am really, suddenly, on this cloud with my poem on many levels, about being born and dying, about being afraid and angry, and about eloping into no responsibility, and about loving myself. I don't know what to do first: write or sleep. I can't believe yet that it is over. That Rachel is off.

And I miss her. I miss the adrenaline and perhaps the hate. And I miss being better than I am.

❦　❦　❦

Paul had complained when Rachel was a freshman. He was not seeing her frequently enough. Rachel said nonsense, she saw him when she had to. Through the Foundation, which occupied more and more of Mark's time, he met an excellent physician from Providence who was deeply involved with the disease. We suggested to Rachel that she see him if she did not always want to make the trip to New York. But she wouldn't hear of it. Paul, reviled all those years as insensitive, was now the only one she trusted, the only one who wasn't trying to destroy her existence, who treated ulcerative colitis as an illness, not a way of life; he kept her going; he understood.

I said to Mark that I thought that she was being a heroine for Paul's benefit, that there was some lack of communication.

"What do you mean?"

"She told me the other day that at the end of a consultation, Paul said that now he'd have to go see his *sick* patients. I tried to explain that this had been a little joke, but she was taking it literally. Paul doesn't consider her sick; he'd be disappointed if she made a fuss; he knew she could take it, that she wouldn't give in, that she'd keep going. You know, all that."

"There's truth in that."

"But being his star isn't worth withholding information."

"Does she do that?"

"It's hard to say. The whole business of her exercising her judgment about what is important and what isn't. I've heard her say a number of times that this or that isn't worth telling him, "has nothing to do with it," or that Paul would laugh at her."

"Does he?"

I had to smile. "You know his humor; it's not always clear. No, more often I think the problem is that Rachel will report something and Paul will merely nod, not comment. Then she interprets that to mean that it was too unimportant to merit discussion; next time she won't mention it."

"More likely he doesn't comment to avoid one of her endless arguments if he doesn't prescribe exactly what she thinks he should. I'm really beginning to see what he means when he says that she's depriving herself of optimal care."

"I don't know!" Suddenly I felt defensive for her, angry at both Mark and Paul. They wanted it both ways, didn't they? She had to be Supergirl, but also submissive as all hell! I said sharply, "It probably doesn't make the slightest damn difference except to help her tolerate an impossible situation. Let her have the feeling that she's in charge of something!"

Mark nodded; he really wasn't the enemy. He said, "You're right. And basically she manages incredibly well."

On and on we went, until we had talked ourselves back into thinking that all was well in this best of all good worlds. And perhaps it was, under the circumstances.

Later that year Rachel's language became unintellgible to us. And just to heft some of the books she was studying seemed unreal. Opened at random, the text yielded nothing I could understand. She, however, though dissatisfied with her first semester's grades, did seem to grasp content and concept.

I think it was around that time that we first began to be scared about chromosome mutation. It was not quite clear how the worry had crept in; certainly nothing in my daily life touched on such matters. But Rachel lived in a medicine-related world now; spoke to lots of people—older students, professors, also fellow freshmen who fancied themselves most knowing. The first thing I remember hearing was that 6-mercaptopurine worked by interfering with nucleid acid biosyntheses and that some doctor had called it mutagenic. It sounded horribly scary to me, and I wasn't sure whether Rachel was just showing off with her big words or whether she used that cool scientific tone to cover a fear of her own.

I asked Paul, who seemed surprised about the question but then answered readily enough. Yes, in a review paper he and Dr. Dash had done there was a reference to a case Leb discusses in which he was able to demonstrate chromosomal abnormalities in the mother as well as the newborn after the mother had received the drug during pregnancy to prevent rejection of a transplanted liver. Why? Was Rachel planning to have a baby just then?

We laughed. No, Rachel had enough worries about her bio grade; she wasn't experimenting with the real stuff. And as the conversation turned to other matters I sat, dissatisfied, still unknowing. What *had* Paul said? But did not dare to go back to the subject and insist on clarification. Instead I put it on the back burner for the time being.

Sometime afterward, the Foundation brought out an excellent pamphlet titled "Some Frequently Asked Questions About Pregnancy in Ileitis and Colitis." And there it was, very clearly: "Question: Should immunosuppressive drugs such as Imuran and 6-mercaptopurine be used during pregnancy? Answer: Once the pregnancy has been diagnosed, immunosuppressive drugs should not be started because of the potential genetic damage to the fetus. If conception occurs while a woman with ileitis or colitis is being treated with immunosuppressives, termination of pregnancy can be justified." Reading that, I was satisfied that the problem was simply one to face if and when Rachel would want to have a child. No immediate concern, blinders firmly in place. Even though Paul once more attempted to take Rachel off the drug during that year. However, she relapsed badly again and had to be put back on it.

I remember that Mark and I, while not actually hiding it, did avoid showing the pregnancy pamphlet to Rachel. Our stated reason was that she had all she could handle, and since it wasn't an acute problem, why burden her? What we didn't face then, or even much later, was the worry about whether these drugs could produce damage in a young woman prior to pregnancy, whether someday we might be in for a horrible surprise. And what we obviously couldn't tolerate at all was to find out that Rachel was walking about with such worries.

During most of that year, Rachel was exhausted. "We should have *made* her defer acceptance at Brown for a year!" I said to Mark. "Look how well she did in Israel!" The thought, always lurking—how much of an influence did the school pressure have on the state of her health? But these thoughts did not stand up to examination, because in Israel she had also filled her life to the brim, had also taken on undue amounts of responsibility. It was her nature, and perhaps she needed the satisfactions this way of life produced more than the leisurely pace I kept urging her to take. And there were satisfactions. In the science courses she had managed to do some of the work she enjoyed and did best. A paper written as a lab requirement for biology, titled "When Medical Technology Fails," was recommended for publication in the *Rhode Island Medical Journal* by her professor. She called to tell me, obviously pleased but also a little afraid. "Send it to me," I said, thrilled for her.

It was a good paper, and it was again a paper in protest against the American way of death. She started it with the quote from Ecclesiastes: To everything there is a season. Oh, yes, a season to live and a season to die; when would Rachel have a season to be carefree? It made me cry, but Mark comforted me when he pointed out to me that her ability to control her fears by intellectualizing them was obviously her method of coping. Just the same, the next time we had an opportunity to speak quietly by ourselves I did suggest that she might now benefit by some psychological counseling, that perhaps she was carrying too heavy a burden. Her answer came easily; it was obviously neither an outrageous nor a surprising thought—no, not now: "I couldn't cope with that now."

In the late fall Paul asked her whether she would like to take part in a T.V. interview the Foundation would have on the ABC network, on *A.M. America*. He explained that there would be approximately fifteen minutes, minus time for commercials, during which he'd like to give a quick medical overview of the disease, have the founder of the organization explain its function and purpose, and have Rachel speak about her life-style as a patient, student, and young person who was not being stopped by the disease. "Think about it," he suggested.

Over Thanksgiving we had a lot of discussions. Sam, of course, was completely opposed. Why should she expose herself like that? Go on T.V., tell the world that she has diarrhea! Nuts!

"That's not the way I see it," she came back heatedly. "I can help someone who's just getting sick, who's scared, who doesn't know whether it's going to spoil their life. I can say to them that it's manageable."

"That's utter nonsense. First of all, because you can hack it doesn't mean that this other person can; everyone's case is different."

"You're both right," I intervened. Anyhow, it was inevitable for Rachel to do this, if for no other reason than because Paul had chosen her from among his patients. It confirmed to her that she held the coveted place of the patient who was responding to his medical management, that she had grown and developed satisfactorily, that she was proof that his theories worked; it was a way in which she could give Paul a magnificent present. I could also see, but not say to the children, that the whole idea represented a challenge to Rachel, a testing of herself and all the times she had argued for facing hard facts, the very ideas she expounded in her papers on the care of the dying: the principle of facing the truth and accepting it. It seemed to me that there was no way that she could crawl out of her commitment to these ideals. And I wished that Sam would stop badgering her, even though, emotionally, I shared his view. Why did it have to be Rachel who had to sacrifice her privacy? Why not some other kid? Why not Judi?

An advertisement the Foundation had placed in two leading papers recently had shown a girl of perhaps twelve, a thin child, a child the camera caught in a pose that tore into me with its truth— her head lowered, her hands clasped to her belly: a child in pain. The caption said, JUDI HAS A TUMMY ACHE THAT MAY NEVER GO AWAY. I had stared at it, too hurt to cry, too moved to resent the exploitation underneath: GIVE TILL IT STOPS HURTING! Oh, very fine P.R. Only, did it affect people who didn't have the intimate knowledge of Judi's gesture? And now they would exploit Rachel. I said to Sam, who was still arguing, "Shut up, Sam. It's Rachel's decision."

We ate turkey and all the trimmings. Later we walked at the beach, Mark and I leisurely, Rachel jogging, Sam sprinting ahead. Between Mark and me it needed little discussion. He summarized it absolutely when he said, "I wish Paul hadn't asked. But I guess it was inevitable."

In spite of our certainties, however, Rachel took time deciding. Whatever the forces were that we thought of as "inevitable," there were also strong countercurrents. At last, a couple of weeks later, it was Paul who told us that she had called to say she would do it.

We were much more satisfied with the image, the time, the attention the Foundation was getting now. The seventh annual dinner would have a fund-raising goal of half a million dollars, and the best news was not just the good P.R.—Monte Hall had just done a T.V. spot for us—but the fact that excellent doctors were associating themselves with the effort. Dr. Baldwin from Mayo would be honored at the dinner; Dr. Ashbrook of Boston and Harvard and Massachusetts General Hospital would head the grants-review committee. In the long run, that was the most important, the only, hope: enough money, enough talent, enough time (enough time for Rachel?) to find the cause and cure.

The actual event—Rachel's appearance on T.V.—was probably bound to be emotionally anticlimactic. I had been upset and nervous in anticipation. Rachel claimed that she was not. And then there she was on the tube, speaking intelligently, but unable to get her point across because the interviewer insisted on asking questions that were not pertinent and time was short. Paul, on the other hand, having more uninterrupted time, was able to say his piece—a mini explanation of ileitis and ulcerative colitis and a maxi push in delivering a not very subliminal message: it's no disgrace to have diarrhea, you're not alone, go for help!

Before Rachel rushed back to school, she expressed her disgust at the waste of time it had been. "The whole point I wanted to make . . . to say that it doesn't have to stop you . . ." She shrugged. "Oh, well!" She raced the motor, impatient. I kissed her through the window. "At least," I said, "at least they saw a beautiful girl who goes to a good college; that's a message in itself."

"Like fun!"

She was angry, I saw. At me (why hadn't I stopped her?), at Paul ("Boy, the way he said d-i-a-r-r-h-e-a"), at the situation. Later, with more perspective, she poked fun at herself, "And I really thought I'd be making a contribution, that my sacrifice would not be in vain. . . ."

❧ ❧ ❧

The smelly cat had disappeared. Ruth, thinking that Rachel was heartbroken, bought her a new one. But the truth was that Rachel neither needed nor wanted a cat in her college setup. It was quite a dilemma, and not easy for Rachel to say, Thank you, but no, thank you, to Ruth, who was able to return the little creature to the pet shop. I was very much pleased with the incident—Ruth being so loving, Rachel making a noncompulsive judgment. It was one of those small occurrences that suddenly made me brimmingly aware that my children (Ruth firmly included now) were marvelous.

And then came the next exacerbation, fouling up the spring term. But Rachel stayed up at school and struggled through. She doctored with Paul over the telephone. Yes, yes, she knew it was time for x-rays and a biopsy; as soon as the exams were over she would come. "You'll see, she'll only go to him the day before he takes off on his vacation!" I predicted angrily to Mark.

"So what? Don't push her now because of a week or two."

"You don't understand. That means that I'll have to worry all summer about the biopsy. If she'd go sooner, it would be back before he leaves, and I'd have a carefree summer. But no! And why? Just to do it *her* way."

"If anything bad showed up in the biopsy, whoever covers for Paul would pick it up," Mark soothed.

I tried to be satisfied with that. "Anything bad!" Oh God, we were approaching the dreaded ten-year mark. In all the literature, that was the witching hour—the time of a heightened peril of malignancy. We had read all kinds of different percentage rates, but on one thing all the authorities agreed: after ten years of active ulcerative colitis . . .

And I had known my Rachel well; she did indeed postpone the ordeal to the last minute. Then, with it past, she began a happy summer of work at Mt. Sinai Hospital. Her co-workers in the lab were very congenial; everyone was premed. And there were the concerts in the park and opera and tennis at lunchtime. Free in New York; I was in the country, where Rachel showed up weekends. And a boyfriend with a beard, Peter, also a premed student.

I don't know why Mark's prediction that someone would pick up any irregularity in the lab report of Rachel's biopsy did not prove to be right. It must have been because the irregularity was minor. That's what I kept saying to myself and Mark in the ten days it took to get the new biopsy back. But minor or not, it caused Paul, on his first day back from vacation, to find Rachel at her job at Mt. Sinai and ask her to come in so that he could repeat the test.

When I saw her that weekend, she said that Peter had insisted on going with her, which indicated to me how frightened she must have been. Obviously, they had done a lot of talking, these doctors-to-be, undoubtably filled with the zeal of little knowledge, perhaps scaring themselves silly. Or perhaps just more realistic than I dared to be. In any case, for the first time in all those years of dealing with ulcerative colitis, the word "cancer" was mentioned between Rachel and us. Rachel saying, "If I have cancer . . ." in a tentative tone, Mark interrupting with an explosion, "Rachel!" and I, sharply, "Stop talking nonsense!" Then we were quiet, hearing the hum of the motor. We were on our way to the city. It was Monday morning. Rachel and Mark had to go to work; I had an appointment with my editor.

All that week, back at the beach by myself, living with mounting terror, I reproached myself for this incident. Rachel had wanted to talk; we had cut her off. Obviously she was beginning to face alternatives now. In a long telephone conversation, Paul had been very reassuring. He said that the likelihood was that the cell irregularity that had appeared in the biopsy report would prove to be nothing—"A laboratory mistake; you don't know how often this happens!"—but that even if it was still there, it would indicate only a precancerous condition, a situation that would suggest the advisability of considering elective surgery. "Elective!" he emphasized; there would be no emergency forcing us into hasty decisions.

Over the years of Rachel's illness we told ourselves again and again that her pain, the restrictions on her life, the discomforts she suffered were in the cause of avoiding surgery. And Paul's repeated statements that she was not a candidate for surgery had upheld us. But now we had to give Rachel an opportunity to explore how she felt about the possibility of surgery.

Thoughts tumbled like the breakers at my feet as I stood staring out over the ocean. What about the new procedure I had heard of, an ileostomy that did not require the wearing of an appliance? Was it still too experimental? And thoughts intruded while I was trying to do revisions on my new book, and I found that now, in my unconscious, there was a ready-made idea that I had never had before: maybe it's just as well to get it over with, because sooner or later, when Rachel wants children, she will have to opt for the surgery first anyhow. And more thoughts over the clatter of the typewriter: maybe it would be a relief for her not to live with the constant dread of malignancy? I jumped up, began to pace. No, no, who said that Rachel lived with that fear? I was projecting, letting my own hysteria overwhelm me. It was not for me to talk, to suggest, to comment. What I had to do was listen, listen to Rachel, *find out* what she was thinking.

I called her on Thursday and apologized for having cut her off on Monday morning when she had wanted to talk. I said, "Let's sit quietly this weekend and discuss it." And maybe, I thought, maybe the test will be back tomorrow and all the worry laid to rest. . . .

Rachel replied, her tone noncommital, "Monday morning? I don't remember." Then, "Hey, I'm bringing Peter and Liza out. Is that okay?"

"Sure," I said. "Sure." Hanging up, I thought that there was no better way to barricade yourself against a "talk" than company. Oh, well, there was no way for me to face this ultimate conversation with Rachel prepared, anesthetized, intellectually alert; it would simply hit me one day, out of the blue, at Rachel's choosing. And I'd better not run again when it did.

Lots of laughter Friday night and Saturday morning. Peter, Liza, and Rachel in the small sailboat in a brisk wind, capsizing into the warm water, shrieks of delight. Mark and I, by the shore, watched them. Then I heard the phone and ran back to the house. "Jean?" Paul's resonant voice. "I was just going to hang up; I thought you weren't home."

"I had to run up from the pond." My heart pounding.

"I've just come from the lab. I didn't want you to have to wait till Monday if the tests were ready. They were. They're okay, absolutely perfect. Active ulcerative colitis, nothing else!"

I burst into tears and handed the phone to Mark, who had come up behind me.

Still, the subject had been broached. And it seemed to me that Rachel was provoking—or perhaps the word was "inviting"—me to talk of the surgery. One day, in the car again, and protected against real debate by one of her endless succession of houseguests, she said apropos of her plans for some activty, ". . . and if Paul takes me off the six-MP again and it doesn't work, he'll just have to put me back on."

"He might not always be able to do that," I protested.

"Well, there's no other alternative," she answered sharply. Then waited.

I said that was not true, aware of the weakness of my reply. But we were in the presence of a stranger; I felt that Rachel was counting on my reticence.

On another day she braved it when we were alone. Again maneuvered to the jump-off point, I did say that the reality of the situation was that an alternative did exist.

Her voice frightened, she asked, "What?"

"You know I'm talking about the surgery, Rachel."

"That's ridiculous." An angry laugh. "That's completely out of the question."

I said no more. Why did she have to put me into this position? I felt torn, angry, and confused. Making a clumsy gesture, I knocked the coleus we had just repotted to the floor. Dark soil scattered all over the kitchen. I yelled, Damn, then leaned my head against the kitchen cabinet, fighting for control. Rachel, without a word, started sweeping up. By the time I had myself together, she was done. I thanked her, but she shook her head as if saying, Don't be silly. It was a sudden reversal of roles, oddly comforting for me.

Mark and I talked endlessly. What was going on? Was there an inner process, a preparation, a test taking place in Rachel? And what was our part to play? What role was she assigning to us? It reminded us a little of the way she had sometimes provoked us when she'd been small. Blatantly naughty, she had sent out messages that she wanted to be stopped. But now she wasn't three years old. Now she had to come to her own peace, her own decisions; we daren't inject ourselves. "We have to be as nonmanipulative as possible," I warned Mark.

"Considering that I don't even know what I myself think or feel, never mind what I want, how can I manipulate? All I know is that I hurt."

"We manipulate," I said. "We send signals."

"What kind?"

"I don't know. That's what worries me. I know we mustn't."

The weekend Sam came back from Washington, where he had worked as an intern for a Senator, Peter was there as well. I realized that regardless of the amount of bickering that went on between brother and sister, there was no doubt that Sam was the one against whom all male creatures were measured. Rachel had been furious that he'd never taken any of her other conquests seriously. Furious, I think, because it influenced her. So when Sam and Peter went running along the beach together on Sunday morning, I said, "Sam likes this one in spite of his going to Harvard."

Rachel, helping me make breakfast, shrugged. "Ivy League jerks!" she said. "Jocks! Peter is going out for crew—would you believe it?"

"Well, they are not exactly stupid," I defended.

"Peter is very immature. Except, he's science-smart." Her voice still pretending contempt.

"You'll be glad enough to know him next year when he can help you with organic chemistry."

Then she burst into a fantastic laugh; the truth was, she was happy. And I was crazy about Peter.

CHAPTER 11

"When Mom and Dad came up to Providence last fall to celebrate my 20th birthday, we were a little hard put for a real celebration. I'd all but stopped eating at that point already but I didn't want them to realize. So we dined like royalty that night; I was sick for days after that.

Rachel, May 28, 1977

JUNE 17, 1977

It is a year and a month today since Sam's commencement at Yale: May 17, 1976. It was perhaps the last marvelous moment we had before all the trouble started in earnest. I think of it today, of what we went through in that baker's dozen of months; I think of it—only a year older?—from that happy day to this lovely afternoon. Earlier I picked up Rachel at the plane from Providence, and just a few moments ago she came to my room to model the dress she will be wearing on Sunday when we go to the garden wedding of the daughter of close friends. A dress of white cotton lace, and green lizard sandals with high heels, and Rachel executing a pirouette, her hair swinging after her.

I have a sense that time is telescoping, the past and present slipping one within the other: clear-walled cylinders containing fate like water. It interferes with perspective, perhaps, but feels so alive. I smell the heat, the worry in the crowd about Rachel on crutches but also the eagerness pushing me forward to see, to watch, to find Sam in the snake of graduates. It was a brilliant day, and Sam was graduating magna cum laude, and I thought, You don't know with what magnificent excellence, how he has overcome. I pushed the hot tears around my cheeks and sniffed and sniffled, and Mark's arm around my shoulders tightened more and more as it got to him too. Oh, not least of all the thought of the venerability of this institution—the sense of time, of history. Next to that, what was the peril of a pair of crutches in the crowd and hauling a little grandma from Kiev, Russia, through the masses, or being in the peristalsis of a mob? A good mob, of course.

The best time was that night at dinner. All our children and Grandma and a favorite cousin. Something of the feeling that we truly loved one another. Dan and Rachel celebrating Sam's day without reservation. Sibling problems, any problems, laid aside for one perfect moment of unity. Almost drowning in beatitude, I thought that it was all worth it.

❦ ❦ ❦

Rachel's sophomore year was an improvement in all but her state of health. She was living in the Grad Center in a pleasant single room, her plants were flourishing, her kitchen—half a closet behind a curtain—was one of the wonders of the world, and she had lots and lots of friends. The only problem seemed to be an overabundance of goodies at the start of the year when to Peter at Harvard was added a Len at Brown. For a while I think that Rachel believed she could balance it—have her pie and eat it too. But the dilemma was apparently solved by the fact that Len was a proponent of commitments and deep relationships; Rachel still felt unable to make promises of this sort. It was take it or leave it—friendship. Len "took" being a friend and is still a terrific one. So, more and more, I'd hear that Rachel was in Boston (No, she hadn't had time to see the children) or that Peter was in Providence. So it was Peter? Well, yes and no. Rachel still insisted that he was immature, had a temper, was opinionated; she didn't like the way he drove the car: recklessly.

"Doesn't sound like a great love to me," I said to Mark, disappointed.

He thought it was funny. "The way you were projecting, thinking that it's going to rain stars the moment Rachel falls in love. These days they don't suspend judgment for love."

I said, with my somewhat tattered dignity pulled around my shoulders, that it would have been nice for her to have something happy to balance her troubles. Though she said that she was happy enough, they had fun. But mostly, if I asked, she'd say, "Well, we had to be in the library, we worked." The damn premedism.

The appearance of the *Rhode Island Medical Journal* in December 1975 with Rachel's article in it was an event that passed unheralded by trumpet blasts; in fact, she wouldn't even cash in on it when it turned out that one of her professors was a fellow contributor. "Did you point it out to him?" I asked. "Of course not," she answered indignantly. No, the important thing about it was that it would be recorded for all eternity in the *Index Medicus* for anyone to look up. "My first!" she said. And of course, it would be mentioned in her transcript—everything that might possibly look good to a medical-school admissions officer was getting crucial. Yet she was up against the old numbers game: how to get grades and still take courses that interested her, and how to have a major that was both of her choosing and a suitable preparation for medical school. When she came up with something called "Biomedical Ethics Concentration," it smacked to me of more of Rachel's independent-project stuff; but the school did recognize it as a legitimate major, and Rachel settled into courses in the religious studies, philosophy, and science departments.

Because of her work in thanatology she obtained permission to take a course called "Living with Dying" which was under the medical-school faculty. The professor who taught it became a close friend. His wife, Olivia Bradshaw, was a nurse; Douglas, a physician. Rachel had in common with them an acquaintance with suffering and illness: Olivia had lost a child to cancer; Douglas, an arm. And I think that they were also drawn together by their ability to survive. Rachel's respect for Doug originated, not least of all, on the tennis court; he beat her handily.

When the snows came, I was glad that she had the big old Lincoln up at school; it had good tires. Both children complained (and Sam had absolutely refused to take it to New Haven, while Rachel felt that it was better than no transportation at all in Providence) that it felt as if they were riding around in a fortress in that car. Which was exactly what made it the perfect vehicle as far as I was concerned. I called Rachel one Sunday afternoon when it was coming down hard around New York and found her at Peter's. "Do stay put," I said. "The radio says the storm is moving in your direction."

She answered that she had to get to the library at Brown, that it wasn't snowing there as yet, and that they could probably beat it. "Peter should be back from the lab any moment; then we'll leave right away."

We next heard from her some hours later after the car had crashed into a guardrail. "I think it's totaled," she cried. "Damn Peter." And after a pause, "Poor Peter, he feels terrible."

We ascertained that neither of them was hurt and told them to put the matter into Dan's lawyer hands; they were still in the Boston area. Which they did, and then took the train to Providence.

Dan, very properly, called up his garage and had the car towed to the body shop he himself used. After a few days, Mark asked me whether the car had been seen by an insurance adjuster and what its status was. I said that I hadn't inquired; considering that our-son-the-lawyer was handling the matter, I hadn't wanted to exhibit any pushiness. "I mean, just because he's the kid who put his burning pipe into the glove compartment when he was sixteen!" Mark laughed; Dan had never lived that one down. But after another week, I did ask on the telephone—very casually—"Say, Dan, what ever happened to the Lincoln?"

"The Lincoln?" he asked. "Ah yes, the Lincoln! I hoped you wouldn't ask."

"What's the matter?"

"Well, at present the car has disappeared."

I burst into wild laughter. Totaled and stolen!

"And I wanted to impress Dad with my efficiency!" he moaned before joining my laughter.

Eventually the car reappeared as the snow melted; it had only been buried in a drift in the lot of the body shop. That had been a bad storm. Also eventually it got fixed. The only trouble was that it took three months—which, however, suited me fine; I hated for Rachel to drive in bad weather. Nor did she mind either; the accident, the sickening lurch, the sense of being out of control had left her without the appetite to do more winter driving. Because she blamed herself for the accident.

"But you weren't even driving, and anyhow, it was pure ice and the snow was blinding Peter." I protested.

"I know, but I should have put my foot down. When Peter was so late coming from the lab, I should have insisted that we stay. I told him we should, that I didn't want to drive. He said not to be silly, he would drive." She looked at me. "You see? That's what I mean about Peter!" Then she repeated, "But I should have put my foot down."

I understood. The charming boy, the intelligent one, the stubborn male pride . . . I'll drive—famous last words; difficult to handle without being very rough. Certainly difficult for as young a woman as Rachel. And if he was that way in other matters as well . . .

"Yes, I see," I said.

There is a picture of Rachel that Peter took in the yard of Lowell House at Harvard. It shows her wearing a knitted parka which Mark had brought her from Copenhagen. With one hand she holds on to a thick tree branch, her body is curved unselfconsciously, she is laughing, and her hair is whipping in the wind; I knew that it wasn't all that bad.

I don't really remember how the research project had its original start. I think it evolved out of conversations Douglas and Rachel had in connection with the work they did—Rachel's growing interest in thanatology, Douglas' specialization in lung diseases, their mutual involvement in the "Living with Dying" course. The first time I heard of it, there was already talk that Rachel would get some funding, and that it would be she who'd have to devise and/or adapt the psychometric instruments for testing a group of terminally ill respiratory patients.

The purpose was to compare their locus of internal versus external control, their profiles of mood states, and their quality of life while dying, with studies made on cancer patients. Douglas had brought a third person into the study, a Dr. Adam Truman who was a psychologist; Rachel would work with and under him. She would stay in Providence the following summer to commence the project, which would, however, flow into the following year, since it was their intention to observe the patients over an extended period of time (or until their death, whichever came first) and, hopefully, to be helpful in their care. Indices would be compiled measuring depression, anger, hope, vigor, fatigue, confusion, and bewilderment. Rachel would write her honors thesis on the subject, and the study would provide knowledge that would be a contribution to the care of terminal patients.

We were a little overwhelmed by the seriousness of it all. We also doubted that anyone as young as Rachel, even if and after she had concocted some wonderful psychometric instruments, could do these interviews. Mark said to her, "Suppose I'm dying of T.B. I'm fifty-seven years old, I'm scared, I'm weary. And you walk in and toss your hair back and start to ask me questions. I think I'd say to you, 'What the hell do *you* know?' "

"I'd answer, 'I know nothing. But I'd like to listen if you'd tell me.' "

We were at the dining-room table. I watched Mark and Rachel, who were facing each other with great intensity. At her answer, the tension left Mark's face, his mouth relaxed; it was a crumpling into softness, acceptance. "Yes," he said and nodded. "Yes, I'll talk to you."

Dramatic stuff, a moment during which Mark had completely projected himself into being that desperately sick man. And a moment when all three of us understood fleetingly how deep the need for communication is and how desperately lonely it is to die. I also knew suddenly that Rachel was speaking from experience when she explained about the isolation of being sick. She had recently written that the specific fear of dying was secondary to the more devastating dread of desertion, annihilation, and alienation. At that moment, while she and Mark stared at each other, I felt in my heart that these matters, these interests, these morbid-seeming preoccupations were Rachel's answer to her own mortal fear. If she could be instrumental in helping someone else accept a dreaded reality, it was in the service of her own fight against denial. Or did she use this psychic energy in helping others to have none left for herself? And who could tell? And even if I understood, what could I do?

There was the business of the accidents. The previous year Rachel had spent some time on crutches as a result of a freak accident. While looking for something that had rolled beneath her bed, she had dropped the bed on her foot. In the family, we compared that one to a neighbor's broken neck suffered as she fell into the garbage can.

Now, this year, Rachel fell out of a liquor store. Peter was coming, they would go dancing; she had hurried home from class, then remembered that she had promised one of her suitemates to bring a bottle of wine. Carrying it and her books, she tripped on some uneven steps leading down from the door and fell, holding the bottle aloft, not breaking it. They spent that evening at the hospital, and then Rachel was back on crutches. When I saw her some weeks later, the *good* leg, the one not in the cast, still had the most god-awful bruises.

I remember, looking at it, that I had a feeling of despair. With one exacerbation running into the next, with all these accidents, it was as if luck had run out, and that we were walking into some tragedy. Yet, I told myself, there was the counterbalance of good things: Rachel's excellent marks that year, her friendships, the esteem in which both the Drs. Bradshaw and Truman and their wives held her, and the respect Mark and I felt for her too. Still, more and more, there was a sense of being blind; weren't we simply standing at the bottom of a hill waiting for a truck to come roaring out of control into our midst?

During the summer we didn't see much of Rachel. She came for a couple of weekends, always with friends; behind her moat. She was tanned but tired-looking. Together with a friend, she was house-sitting for a professor. Yes, they got along all right. Was she seeing Peter? Not lately, but she told me in June that he'd taken her to hear the annual *1812 Overture* in the yard of Lowell House. It was lovely. "You know they have this bell tower, and they ring their bells at the very moment Tchaikovsky's score calls for them." Yes, yes, but how did she feel? Okay. What did that mean? She said sharply, "What do you want? Exact descriptions? Bloody mucosa, thin stools, cramps, backaches, pain in my joints?"

"Is that how it is?"

More calmly, "Sometimes."

The only subject to which she warmed was her relationship with the Trumans and the Bradshaws. "You must meet them, Mom; you'll love each other." And the progress of the project—the questionnaires were ready, the criteria set, the psychometrics established.

One evening Rachel and I walked down to the pond. In a sky still bright, a pale moon was waiting. We watched the last covey of birds land and disappear into the reeds, saw the waters ripple, then calm, as the light faded. All the time the moon was gaining in color and shine, and when the pond was finally dark gray velvet, the moon laid a silver swath upon it. I longed to say many things: that I was observing that Rachel hardly ate anything, and I wanted to ask whether she was not due for x-rays, and when had she last seen Paul? And what was the matter between Peter and her? But I hated to break the serenity of the moment.

It was Rachel who suddenly said, "I guess I'll make an appointment with Paul pretty soon; it's driving me crazy to think of all the junk I'm ingesting."

I answered passionately, sluice gate opened, "You know Paul's been waiting to take you off!" We both knew what "junk" she meant. "It's you who always put off going . . ."

"I didn't have time."

"But Rachel—"

"Skip it, Mom." She put her arm around me to make up for the abruptness. Then said, her voice tired, "You know, some days it's not so bad. Then I think I'm imagining the whole thing."

Rachel was very gentle with me for the rest of the weekend, but she kept the subject off herself.

"Take care of yourself," she said as we hugged good-bye.

"If you promise to eat."

"It's a deal."

We smiled at each other with some irony; it was clear that neither of us knew whether we could stick to these commitments.

Right after the Jewish holidays Paul took Rachel off the 6-mercaptopurine. He said that he could no longer justify its use, especially since it did not keep the lid on anymore. He increased the ACTH dose and suggested trying the Azulfidine once again. Rachel was to start with a small amount, which she was to increase until she was taking twelve a day if they agreed with her. After listening, I asked, "What is she to do if she is in bad pain?" I felt I had to raise the point, since Rachel was obviously not going to say anything. She was just sitting there, her face closed up. But then she surprised me and added, "Yes, and what about the pain in my legs?"

Well, Darvon, of course. Rachel replied angrily that Darvon didn't do a blessed thing for her. So Paul prescribed another pain-killer to take if necessary. And, if necessary to control the running, a few drops of opium. I cringed at each "if necessary." Telling Rachel "if necessary" meant to her that she was not to take it. A million arguments stretching into the past: I saying, "Take something, please," unable to bear the sight of her rolled into a ball of pain, pushing the sweat-soaked hair out of her face, pleading,

"Paul said you could." And she, "No, it's not necessary." It seemed to me that Rachel could not measure what was necessary.

As we were discussing it on our way home, she shrugged, then rummaged in her bag and brought out a crumpled drawing. "Here, that's Lenny's version of it," she said.

At the next red light I studied it:

The Rachel Bergman/Normal Person
Pain Conversion Scale

Increasing Pain	Person		Rachel	Increasing Discomfort
	Major Disaster	—	—Medium	
	Catastrophe	—	—Moderate Discomfort	
	Major Pain	—	—Mild Discomfort	
	Mild Pain	—	—	
	Threshold of pain—		—	

"Funny?" Rachel asked.

"Not very," I replied.

In the morning I took her to the airport; school was starting. She said that she was pessimistic. "It's never worked without the six-MP before." And just before boarding, "He's got to put me back." When I came home, I understood her anxiety better. In her bathroom there was still the faint odor of blood.

Mark and I had a long telephone conversation with Paul that evening. He repeated to Mark why he had to take her off the 6-MP, but he said again that, while she was having another exacerbation, the x-ray he had taken yesterday did not indicate that she was a candidate for surgery. In fact, the right side, the ascending colon, did not look all that bad, though the descending, the left side, and the transverse colon appeared active right now. He said, "Let's wait for the biopsy to come back," and that he hoped that the Azulfidine would be helpful; some patients did very well on it. "If Rachel would only take it easy for a while."

"What if the Azulfidine doesn't work?" I asked.

"Let's take it one step at a time."

"She won't take Prednisone," I said, surprising all of us.

There was a second of shocked silence; then the men commenced talking. There was always the Foundation. Mark was treasurer and chairman of the finance committee now; Abe Beame would be honored at the ninth annual dinner dance; close to a million dollars was committed in grants and research projects; and the past year had seen the formation of a research-training awards program. I listened, waiting for one or the other to make fund-raising rhetoric, speak of the cause and cure being found soon; waited with clenched fists, ready to clobber them, either or both, or anyone. Dear God, if Rachel had to go back on Prednisone, back to the mooned face—could she do it? Somehow, she had been able to tolerate the ACTH, but the oral steroid was the *bête noire*, the cause of the intense childhood suffering—Beebee, and being different, and being out of it. . . .

After a while Paul asked, "Jean? Are you still on?"

"Yes."

"Look, she'll be all right."

I answered yes, that I knew that. And felt a wave of love for him. Poor Paul, caught in the misery of his impotence with us. But almost immediately I felt a surge of fury too. Who'd told him to get mixed up with this shitty disease? I laughed; an unplesant sound.

"We better hang up," Mark suggestested. We all said good night.

I started to shop for Rachel's birthday soon after that. I was at Lord & Taylor, at Saks, at Bloomingdale's. I bought and bought, and wrapped each package in colored tissue paper and filled a basket. The birthday had to be special this year. Rachel would be twenty, out of her teens.

A week before the event, Mark asked me what I had gotten for her. I was evasive, feeling ridiculous at having been so extravagant. But he had the same goal in mind. "Let's get her something special; she'll be twenty," he announced.

"The kids wear a lot of costume-jewelry chains; maybe I'll get her a bunch of them," I suggested.

"No. Something good."

Suddenly I was angry. I couldn't trace the source. Was I jealous?

What was wrong with what he wanted? Especially since I had been driven into my own excess by the same desire. Then I suddenly understood. We wanted to give her something special because things were bad. Like the goodies, the funny books and baseball cards, the treats and surprises we had brought the children when they were small and had sore throats. Like Sam's Lionel trains. A bribe: don't cry.

The next day I found a necklace made by Mexican Indians; beautiful work, a peacock with his tail spread and a greenish stone in his eye.

We drove up to Providence with the laundry basket adorned with a broad red HAPPY BIRTHDAY ribbon. Rachel had begun her interviews; she was full of it—the story of two sisters, both terribly sick, who each discussed her sister's need to belittle the seriousness of her condition.

It led into the whole subject of denial. I had a strange sense of unreality as I listened to Rachel discuss the phenomenon with great intelligence and insight, saying that some patients, even after they had been told, cannot accept the seriousness of their plight. Sitting there, I remembered that earlier she had responded in an offhand manner to Mark's question about how she was doing without the 6-MP. "I haven't even the time to think about it," she said. Talking of denial. The strange thing was, Rachel was saying, that even those patients who approached the interview with anxiety or even hostility seemed to relax in the process and talk more and more freely.

"Perhaps it's as if they were in talk therapy," I suggested. "Without the onus of going to a psychiatrist."

"I've thought of that." Rachel nodded.

"How long does an interview take?" Mark asked.

"About forty-five minutes, but some run way over. I let them talk if it seems to be what they want." She was suddenly embarrassed, looked away from us, added, "It's sort of nice. I mean, if I can see that someone feels better when he leaves . . ."

I understood. That was the ideal—to aid by acceptance, by caring; to combat the loneliness; to make dying a part of the life circle. For the first time since Rachel had embarked on the whole project, it seemed right to me. Right for her, and for the people she touched with her sincerity, her love.

In the car, after leaving Rachel at her dorm, when I was feeling comfortable because I could focus on Rachel's important work,

Mark collapsed my Tinker Toy structure. "She isn't feeling well," he said. "It's not working without the six-MP."

Just a couple of weeks after that, about ten days before Thanksgiving, Rachel called and asked me to meet the next Allegheny flight. "I've an appointment with Paul," she said. "He's going to wait for me."

"What is it, Rachel?"

"Mom, I've got to run; Len's driving me to the airport."

The telephone was dead in my hand. I sat down on my bed, felt the shaking start inside, but almost immediately controlled it. Not now, not now.

She was bleeding badly, she said, and her joints were really bad; the pain was—well, she tried to grin at me. "You know, moderate discomfort!" I let her out in front of Paul's office, went to park, did some marketing; I was eager to be there, just to sit in the waiting room, to be near. Oh, but I also wanted to stay away, not know.

Then, when I walked in, it was strangely quiet; after office hours; only Paul's voice on the phone from the back. I chatted with the nurse; I waited. At last Rachel joined me. She had been crying. She had a terrible headache. Paul came out and told her to lie down awhile, wait for the painkiller to work, for her head to ease. She was submissive, beaten; went off to lie down in the x-ray room. Paul told me that she had fought him hard, but that he had to put her back on the Prednisone. For the first time in all those years.

I had known, of course. "How much?" I asked.

"Sixty milligrams."

"Are you going to let her go back to school?"

"No."

Relieved, I nodded.

Then Paul went off and I sat and waited for Rachel, who had fallen asleep. This pleasant room, with Picasso's children dancing ring-around-the-rosy, the graceful legs of antique chairs. How often I had sat here; how much pain, fear, indignation I had felt. But at that moment I felt nothing. Or perhaps a kind of peace. Is that how defeat feels?

I said to Rachel as we were driving home that I was proud of her. Then, immediately, wanted to take the words back. Proud why? Because she wasn't kicking and screaming? And as if she knew my thoughts, she said, "Oh, but I tried! Son of a bitch!" Who? What? I didn't ask. And she continued, talking quietly while the tears coursed down her cheeks, not wiping them, letting them run into her neck: "No choice! He gave me no choice. He said if I didn't take it, he'd put me in the hospital and give it to me intravenously." And when I didn't answer, she said, "I know, I know; he's got no choice either."

I considered saying that he'd get her off it as soon as he could, that at least she'd have the comfort of arresting the attack quickly, that this time she was tall enough not to be turned into a little squirrel and she'd carry the weight better. No, no, no. It was better to keep quiet.

At home we found a vial still full of Prednisone. "It's from way back when," she said, and quickly swallowed the little pills. And suddenly we were calm; it had happened.

She worked steadily during the next days. At least, the timing wasn't too terrible: she was losing only a couple of chemistry classes and one lab; one of her classmates would give her his notes. And she could do the paper for Reli Stu at home. Paul had given her a powder which, mixed with water, made a drink of high nutritive value; that was practically all she had. I also heard the old familiar sprint to the bathroom. And waited; it always took a couple of days until the Prednisone took hold. We didn't discuss it. We talked about going to the shore for Thanksgiving. "Len is coming; is that all right?" she asked.

"Of course."

Sam was annoyed when he heard it. Not because he didn't like Lenny. but because of the statement Rachel seemed to be making, the declaration, that we were not enough for her. "When she's that sick you'd think she'd want her privacy, or at least only have the family around," he said.

I argued with him: "On the contrary, as long as she's with her peers, things are 'normal'—"

"But they are not," he interrupted me.

I ignored what he had said, continued: "And it's hard for her to deal with our anxiety on top of her own. If there's company, we have to behave; we can't hover."

Sam shook his head. He disagreed. He didn't look great either. The first year of law school was no picnic; his apartment in the Village was noisy; he was looking forward to the beach, the quiet, to working in peace, to getting some exercise over the Thanksgiving break; it would be his first time back in Quogue since the summer.

I attempted to soothe him. "Rachel says that Len and she have a lot of work too; it will be quiet." As if that were the point!

"I still think she's weird."

Now I was angry. "Look, don't give her a hard time; Len's a very good friend; she's doing the best she can."

And then, a couple of days later, Rachel started to seek me out, wanted to talk, discuss her worries; it was clear that one of the greatest hardships of being home was missing the Bradshaws. I hadn't realized how much support they had given her as her health deteriorated these last weeks. And it was clear that they had really talked. She told me that they asked her whether she was being influenced toward the surgery by us. I asked, "What did you say?"

"I told them no, that you weren't pushing at all. I think they're a little surprised—*everyone* is—that I've been left on these drugs so long; and you know, the cancer fear."

I nodded.

Rachel went on. "I keep telling them that the surgery is out of the question, that Paul says I'm no candidate. But of course, I worry too."

About the drugs? About cancer? I waited, just said, "Yes."

"I mean, there are two things I know for sure: I want to be a doctor and I want to have a family."

Thinking of the pregnancy pamphlet, wondering what she knew, I finally said carefully, "Well there's no reason why you can't have a family as long as you can tolerate being off the six-MP for the duration of a pregnancy."

"Except that it doesn't look as if I can, does it? Like, he'll have to put me back now! Anyhow, how do I know that my chromosomes aren't already shot to hell? Len said, and Peter too—"

"Look," I interrupted. "Meaning no disrespect to your brilliant friends and their scientific knowledge, but you really ought to discuss all this with Paul, not with the kids. Or anyone."

"I'm not discussing it with 'anyone.' But my friends have opinions, informed opinions. And they care. And I listen. Though, believe me, I'm taking everything with a grain of salt. I know Lenny thinks that he's all-knowing, and even Olivia and Douglas, well, they're probably not quite rational when it comes to cancer fear. You know, overanxious. But still! Still, I'm telling you, Paul's got a lot of balls!"

I said, feeling my way as I spoke, "I don't think I'd be so worried if you'd see Paul regularly. I think I'd trust him to make the right decisions if you did. But he doesn't have enough control when you don't see him for months and months." I stopped. Was what I was saying true? I was chopping cranberries and oranges for the relish; my hands were red. Like hell I wouldn't worry! I thought of the recurring dream I was having in which Paul was the mad scientist! But, I argued with myself, but still, that was just hysteria—intellectually speaking, what I had said was correct. If Rachel would only—

"Well, it's academic." Rachel interrupted my thoughts bitterly. "I've got to see him now."

"Rachel, listen, when this exacerbation is over, perhaps you ought to see someone else. There's Dr. Ashbrook in Boston; it's even easier for you to get to him at Mass General than it is to come to New York."

"No. No, I don't think I'd trust anyone except Paul." She paused, thought a moment, then said, "Anyhow, let's wait and see what the colonoscopy shows." She was scheduled to see a specialist the following day; he would conduct this test. It seemed crazy to do it during an acute exacerbation, but apparently Paul had told Rachel that he wanted it done. And since Paul was away until after Thanksgiving, I couldn't argue with him about it.

We fell silent. Rachel was taking the pulp out of orange halves, cutting zigzags along the borders to make baskets for the relish. An attempt to give the baskets handles had failed, shattered by our impatience; too much trouble. I thought of what she had said, the contradictions: that she trusted only Paul, but that he had a lot of balls. Well, not really a contradiction: the idiom could express admiration. Yet I had had the distinct impression that it contained a dose of mistrust, or at least a question about recklessness. And saying in one breath that she worried about her chromosomes and at the same time insisting that Paul allow her to take the 6-MP again. And the business about the surgery—that it was "out of the question": surely she knew that there could be a moment when no choice existed. It was all subtly dishonest—speaking about the fear of malignancy as if she understood, yet denying it in the same breath: Olivia and Douglas are overanxious, not quite rational. I said out loud, "I really think you must discuss all that with Paul when he comes back." I screwed the Mason jar containing the relish shut; we were trying to prepare ahead for Thanksgiving, since we would get to the shore only the night before. "Shall we take a walk?" I asked.

"No, I'm going to study."

I suddenly realized that she hadn't been away from the house at all except in the car. Not away from the bathroom. So there was no improvement. . . .

In a colonoscopy, a thin cathether is introduced through the rectum into the colon. The doctor can see the inside of the walls, can take photographs, can snip off specimens for biopsy. The advantage of this examination is that it affords visibility that goes far beyond the distance that can be seen through a sigmoidoscope—all the way up through the descending, over on the transverse, and down on the ascending colon. It is done under an intravenous drip of Valium and Demerol; the patient is awake to cooperate but has no sense of time or discomfort. In Rachel's case, she was apparently completely knocked out by the drugs, and we had a hard time waking her up. In fact, a couple of hours after the procedure, with the nurses and the doctor anxious to go home, we were still saying, "Wake up, Rachel. Rachel, wake up." Fortunately, Mark had come along; I could not have gotten her into the car by myself. And even after the ride home, Sam had to practically carry her into the house and up the stairs.

To me, the whole thing was incredibly scary. And on top of it, the examination proved inconclusive. Because Rachel was in an acute exacerbation, she had not been able to take the necessary laxatives to clean herself out completely. But we had supposed that the various enemas, which had yielded only blood, had done the trick, especially since she hadn't eaten any solid food in so long. However, it was impossible for the doctor to complete the examination because he had run into an obstruction of stool. He could therefore give us only half a report, and I rejected any discussion of doing the other half. It seemed to me that she was reacting very unnaturally to the whole thing; that her being so knocked out by the drugs which didn't keep other patients from getting up a half hour later and walking out indicated that Rachel was very much more depleted than anyone seemed to know. I said to Mark that night, "It's because she acts so damn tough; I think to this day Paul doesn't understand how much pain she has. Or for that matter, that she hasn't eaten anything in weeks."

The next day Rachel was up and about, wanting us to tell her about it all, laughing, saying, "Quit your kidding; I didn't!" when

I described her sleepy antics. She remembered nothing after being briefed by the secretary, signing the consent form, and greeting the doctor. "He was nice, wasn't he?"

"Very, very nice," I assured her.

I was uneasy leaving the city with Rachel in this state, but since Paul was not there anyhow, we decided not to change our plans and to spend Thanksgiving in Quogue. Mark shared my concern, but Rachel said we were weird: she was perfectly okay; she wanted to get to the country; she wanted to take a long walk along the beach, see the wild geese, ducks, sea gulls . . .

"Ya, ya," I said, "and the hunters!" It was the season; we hated to hear the popping of guns.

"Bastards!" Rachel said; she loved every damn duck.

It was Len who walked along the beach with me on Thanksgiving. He was very well informed, knew all about the disease; another of his friends was also afflicted. He acquainted me with his ideas—or shall I say, doctrines? He expressed himself very strongly. Things couldn't go on like this, he said; Rachel's control was neurotic denial. "Mrs. Bergman, she's always in this awful pain. And she eats nothing."

"Not in school either?" This hope I'd been having—that she was giving *us* the business, that away from home she was eating better. But Len explained to me that it was because every time she ate anything it started the digestive process, which in turn started the pain.

He was also telling me that it was the Azulfidine which was giving her the headaches—nor sparing me the analysis of what the drug contained and what chain reaction it started in the body. Then, accusingly: "Don't you remember, it affected her that way already when she was a little kid?" And indeed, I suddenly recalled that she used to call them "sinus aches." Oh, God . . .

I was feeling very ambivalent toward Lenny by then. He was telling me that I was permitting my child's illness to be mismanaged. He was also full of caring and concern for her. And his knowledge of the whole history! What hours of talking there must have been between them. The arrogance, though, I felt, in a kind of fury: the damned nineteen-year-old arrogance! What was he pushing for except to prove that her parents and doctors were wrong? Or was he right? And how much influence did he have on

Rachel? And then I thought bitterly: oh, probably not much; no one had. She kept her own counsel.

The wind had picked up, whirled small tornadoes of yellow sand into the breakers. I stopped listening. The frustration of being Rachel's friend must also be great. Yet what choice did she have? Whom could she trust? Not Mommy, Daddy, or God. She had a disease without a cure, a disease that had only a "management."

We came back to the lovely aroma of turkey wafting throughout the house, and the good smell of Caroline's sister's sweet potato casserole. Sam and Rachel had built a fire; Mark had opened the wine. I went to get dressed. Rachel was wearing a peasant blouse and her long skirt. In spite of everything, there was the feeling of anticipation. Perhaps, I thought, the sense of occasion will give us a respite. And Rachel said that she was famished, that she could hardly wait for the first mouthful of stuffing; she would eat today. And finally we were all around the festive table and the turkey oozed juices. Sam said impatiently, "Start carving, Dad." But Rachel wasn't there.

It didn't take long for anxiety to sweep away my cheer. "Let me see what's keeping her," I said, and ran upstairs. She was in her bathrobe on the floor; she was scrubbing her rug. All the windows were open to disperse the smell, her clothes in a bundle by the door. "Let me help you," I said, cold inside with desolation. "Let me throw them in the machine for you." I reached to pick up her clothes, but stopped at the sharpness in her tone. "Don't touch them!" Then, trying to control herself, tightly, "Mother, please go downstairs. I'll be along."

Everyone was on a second helping when Rachel joined us. Except me; the turkey seemed dreadfully dry. But once she was there, smiling, apologizing, saying that she hadn't been able to make up her mind what to wear, I guess I entered into the illusion she was creating. Because, suddenly, I was ravenous. I ate and ate. And tried not to watch Rachel push a forkful of stuffing around her plate.

In the stupor of the aftermath of the meal, sitting on the floor next to Rachel, who was on the couch, I made the mistake that broke her. I reached up and put my arms around her. And that's when she began to cry. I held her tightly, but she could not stop. Until Len came over, and sat down next to me and began to speak to her. I got up then, and he moved into my place. Sam, watching the scene, left the room. His door slammed. Oh, Sam, I thought, what difference does it make who can help her? Just as long as someone does.

Around ten that night, we all had tea and played Scrabble and laughed a lot. But later, in bed, Mark also cried.

CHAPTER *12*

ALSO FROM RACHEL'S POEM:
"AT LAST, THE FOREST A CATHEDRAL."

The child is lost.
Deep in this jungle of thoughts,
tangled emotions,
web of fear.
A forest of words . . .
thicket of unasked questions.
And the chainsaws have started their rasp.

JULY 2, 1977

I'm going to abandon the now/then perspective, write the rest of this account straight. I do not have the strength or heart for fancy devices; I need all my resources simply to tell it. It's strange, the blocks I encounter, the blanks. Was it that Monday after Thanksgiving when Paul said that Rachel had to go into the hospital? I can't remember, have to look into my diary. Considering my recall of events in the far past, conversations coming back, the looks on the children's faces, the odors, feelings, thoughts—ten-year-old bits and pieces, all graphic, all available. But last December, ah, that is hard.

Yes, it was on that Monday that Paul told us he would take the first bed he could get at Lenox Hill Hospital. After we left his office, we went to Bloomingdale's and bought Rachel nightgowns.

And while Rachel shopped in her deliberate fashion, I called Mark at the office; I knew he'd be waiting in terrible anxiety. But he had already spoken to Paul, so he asked me how she felt, had she eaten anything, what was her mood? She was okay, I replied; no, she had neither eaten nor drunk anything. We would be back home in an hour.

"Where are you now?"

Suddenly I was laughing. Oh, probably hysteria, but it did seem funny at that moment. "You won't believe this," I said to Mark when I could. "You really won't believe me, but presently she's trying on every goddamn nightgown in Bloomingdale's."

We bought six. It later turned out that they were all wrong, too warm for the overheated hospital and fever, and some of them had long sleeves; we weren't thinking yet in terms of I.V.s.

There had been only one other hospitalization during Rachel's illness—a very short one in the early days. It had proved so traumatic that later Paul always opted for treating her at home. Rachel and I talked of it as we sat in Admissions, waiting. She told me something about it that I had either never known or forgotten: she told me that the little girl next to her had had a brain tumor and that her doctor had been terribly mean. "He yelled at her. All she did was whimper," Rachel told me; her eyes huge with remembered fright, there in the lobby of Lenox Hill. "I was so scared."

Of course, it was different this time. Rachel was an adult; she was used to hospitals from the other end of the spectrum. Even when she hadn't been in hospitals in her capacity as a helper or learner, she had been a special visitor, one of the few people who knew what to say to a seriously ill person. Apparently hospitals did not render her witless with empathy or fear the way they tend to leave me. Once, a couple of years ago, visiting a friend, I lost Rachel only to find her later down the hall helping a strange man back into bed. Wandering down the halls, interested, curious, she had seen his unanswered light, had gone in and offered her services. All the way home, she had regaled me with his "interesting" medical history.

Watching her as we waited, I thought, no, she isn't scared. Perhaps even relieved, the way I was. At least the immediate problem of the food would be relieved by intravenous feeding. And since the Prednisone hadn't worked—had, amazingly, failed for the first time—she could see the logic of the hospital. I didn't know whether she anticipated deciding, with Paul, how best to proceed in getting this attack under control, or whether the hospital represented letting go of the burden, letting "them" take care of her. I hoped the latter, but did not want to take the risk of asking.

She had a large room. It was on an orthopedic floor rather than a medical one, but it was all Paul could get just then. He said he'd move her when an opening occurred, but later it was decided to let her stay because the situation was good, the nurses nice, and the care she required not beyond the knowledge of the staff. I complained that there was no stream of attractive interns, the only one who came was a girl, and Rachel shook her head at me and said to Mark, "Who would have thought that she'd turn into a Jewish Mother yet?"

We started modestly, with one small hanging plant to balance the intravenous drip, and when the nurses thought it was cute, I felt encouraged and turned the room into a forest. Perhaps that's why all the metaphors in Rachel's poem are sylvan. One thing is certain: the madness with which I decorated was to stem the guilt at my relief. I slept that first night as I hadn't slept in a long time—deeply, sweetly. Though waking was not so good. All very fine that I need not worry about a rupture, a megacolon, or malnutrition, that I need not balance the worry against the conviction that I must let her fly, that I need not sit at home and know her at school in God knew what shape, or even down the hall and running to the bathroom. All very good that hospital meant: safe and, to me at least, that "they" would take on my burden. But already that morning, the relief failed to obscure the real issue: what was next?

Very soon after, I realized that there was no "they." There was Paul, of course. He was simply concerned about bringing the attack under control and would not really be drawn into long-term projections. In the first place, let's stop the bleeding, the pain, the weight loss, and how come she's not mooning on enough steroids to blow up a horse? She was receiving the ACTH intravenously plus oral doses of Prednisone, and there were other substances in the drip (Rachel could, of course, give an exact breakdown of what they were). To me the components of the drip remained vague except on a cause-and-effect basis. The pain in her joints, especially in her knees, was quite severe. But both the disease and the steroids produced these symptoms, so that it was impossible to say exactly what the cause of the pain was. In any case, potassium, to replace that which was being destroyed by the steroids, was one of the goodies added to the drip.

There was also another thing I began to understand very quickly. Rachel would not be pain-free in the hospital. Just as her stoicism had kept her from making herself comfortable when she had been on her own, the fear of megacolon dictated caution with painkillers now. So that we were back to the feeling of fear and uncertainty which had gotten displaced in the first euphoria of relief.

I would arrive in the morning to find her depressed, annoyed with little things, unreasonable. "What am I doing here? I should be in school." It seemed ludicrous to me to have to fight Rachel on the basic issue that she was ill. Instead of playing the classic mother role, as the purveyor of reassurance, the one to say, "It's nothing, Bubeleh," I had somehow been maneuvered into a position of having to remind Rachel that this was a serious matter. A crazy game: she'd report on the x-rays and other tests of the day and tell me what Paul had said and then seek my agreement that it was all nonsense. Yes, well, so what, so I'm still bleeding. One day she said, "But Mom, believe me, there were lots of days when I went to class feeling much sicker than I do now. . . ."

We were trying to understand. It was clear that Rachel was scared but mustn't show it. Did she push me into being the gloom-sayer because she needed, over and over, to be reassured that it wasn't wrong for her to "give in," or was it simply because in all those years there had been emotional bonuses attached to hanging tough and perhaps giving them up was harder than we understood? I again brought up the question of a psychiatrist, and it seemed to me that Rachel was considering it. But in the meantime she kept putting me off; seeing a shrink was one more threat to her hold on the reins. From a practical point of view, those reins meant that she would simply not consider the idea that it might be in order to take some time off. No, she could not, would not interrupt her schooling—the road ahead was long enough as it was, and the research had to go on. The second interview with the first patient group had to be conducted at the right time. "You know, they can't wait around for me!" She had to get back.

I said that I certainly hoped that it would be possible for her to do so, but if it turned out that she didn't have the option . . . Oh, lots of words: find a way to make an inner adjustment, be a little flexible, get yourself in shape.

"I swear I'll sign myself out of here," she threatened.

And then again, there were the days when she was subdued, cooperative, and sad; I didn't like those days any better.

On a Saturday morning when I called first thing, she sounded very upset. She had been in terrible pain in the night; no one had helped her. There had been no authorization in her chart to give her anything for her pain. "Would you believe it, they offered me Tylenol! I kept thinking how much better off I'd be at home, where I could help myself."

"Why didn't you have them call Paul or a resident or someone?"

"They are scared to death to call the attendings. You've got to be dying. Anyhow, it was late."

"But . . ." I was hearing noise in the background, loud voices. "Rachel?" I asked.

"I have to go; they're taking me to x-ray."

Calling Paul; Nina told me that he was already at the hospital, had been called to come. I woke Mark, who was still sleeping; it was only eight o'clock. "Come on, let's get down there; I think something is wrong." I told him about my talk with Rachel and that Paul was already at the hospital.

"Did Nina say that he was called to Rachel?"

"I didn't ask."

"He does have another patient or two, you know!" But he was already half dressed.

Downtown, he let me out of the car while he parked. I willed the elevator to come, rushed along the corridor into Rachel's room. She was chatting on the telephone; she was pale; there was a new bottle, a second one, on the I.V. pole. She was saying, "He called it an incipient megacolon" into the telephone. Then she laughed at something she heard, then answered, "Oh but fast action! When I told my doctor about the pain, boy, that orderly was here awfully quickly to get me down to x-ray." She listened, nodded, said, "Right. Very elegantly, it's called frankfurtering. Yes, a whopping antibiotic."

I sank into the visitor's chair. Well, that was the story. What had she said? Incipient! Did that mean: not really? Just starting? I thought of all I knew about megacolon. That the colon swelled up, its walls indeed becoming as smooth as frankfurters, the skin stretched thin, thin. Terribly dangerous to operate because of the chance of rupture. Oh, God.

And Rachel went on and on with her telephone conversation as if she didn't have a care in the world, crying out happily, "Will you? That's super." I felt as if I were behind Alice's looking glass. At last she hung up, said brightly, "Len's driving down from Providence."

"That's nice," I replied, right back in the game.

Her dad got the story directly. Mark asks a million questions when he gets upset; Rachel answered them patiently, calmly. Then, suddenly, in the middle of one of the medical explanations, she was asleep.

Sitting there, watching her sleep, I wondered how much of her strength was expanded to maintain the control. In case of doubt, she knew more about the dangers of this situation than I. I felt grateful that she was sleeping, that she had a respite from being a heroine and brave and cool about it all.

We held our breaths the next couple of days, even though Paul maintained his positive attitude. Every time we saw him we felt better. The antibiotic was bound to take hold, the swelling in the colon would subside, Rachel would come through this fine. Perhaps the most reassuring thing was Paul's appearance—the forceful step, the immaculate attire without a hint of dandyism, the look of success; he was so solid. The lines in his face had deepened over the years, but he was still young-old just as I had seen him that very first time. Over dinner one evening with him and Nina, in front of a blazing fire, I had a rush of confidence. He knew what he was about; everything would be okay.

But then, later on in bed, out of his magic orb, the doubts! What about the subtle introduction of Steven Grossman's talents? Steve was a young surgeon whom we happened to know because he belonged to our synagogue. Paul had joked that he wasn't holding it against Steve that he was a New Jerseyite and a member of our congregation.

In recall, I saw Paul's face again, the way he had laughed; the fire had cast red shadows that had given his face other hollows, an alien look. And then his expression had sobered; there had been a different sharpness and depth to his eyes; he had said, "Steve's one of the best. Innovative, brilliant." Apropos of what? Yes, and Dr. Grossman had been in to see Rachel too. A social visit, he had said to her; they had discussed the rabbi.

No doubt, Dr. Grossman was "standing by"; Paul had alerted him. He had also alerted us tonight while I was feeling blissful in my trust. Okay, and what else had I missed? Yes, a lot of talk of

Rachel's inability to "let go." I thought resentfully that, suddenly, it was all her fault. Was he saying that if she were just to be a bum, letting herself grow fat and lazy, she'd be well? And what had happened to his pride in her, in his star patient whom he chose to exhibit on T.V. as the living proof that the disease did not disable? At two A.M. I was wandering around the house. From the savior, Paul had turned into the villain. I finally took a tranquilizer and went back to bed. Just before dropping off I understood, fleetingly, what ambivalences Rachel must be feeling toward Paul. It's a terrible thing to need another person so much.

I asked Paul straight out the next time I saw him. "Are you saying," I asked, "that if Rachel would take time off from school, would remove herself from pressure, she could be maintained with —let's say—with only manageable discomfort?" I waited. And when he didn't answer quickly enough, I added, "Because if that's what you're saying, then I think you have to *order* it, demand it!"

He put a hand on my arm. "I can't," he answered. "I don't know that this is so." There was pain in his expression and the familiar melting toward him in myself—it was this integrity in his character which we appreciated. Yet it was also this which placed too heavy a burden of control on Rachel. The fact was that no one knew, that the disease acted erratically and differently in everyone. Sure, all of us—Paul and Mark and I and especially, perhaps, Sam, who was deeply and painfully involved—wanted terribly that she try it. Why not? At twenty, what's a lousy year? Go to Israel, go to the beach, be happy. But yet we all knew that the likelihood was that it wouldn't make much difference. And Paul, being himself, could not assume a pose of "knowing" when, really, he did not; he would not prescribe leisure as a wonder drug. Anyhow, I argued with myself, it was academic. Rachel would not have gone along with us. There was her rage to "get on with it," to learn, to grow, to participate in life. As she was to put it later in her poem: ". . . trembling with desire to be serious about life." No, putting her out to pasture would probably raise pressures far worse than the reality ones.

So we sweated it out. And after a few days Paul told us that the x-rays indicated that the dreaded process had been reversed. "I don't mind telling you, I am relieved," he said.

At which Rachel set up her clamor to go back to school, or at least, to go home. "If I have to," she bargained, "I'll go out to the shore with Mom and do nothing, just rest."

"We'll see," Paul said, maddening her. And when she kept on arguing, he yelled, "Damn it, Rachel, no! Let up."

I hadn't been present during this exchange. Rachel presented it to me in a tone of hilarity. "You should have seen him; he was mad!" But at the same time, she was watching my face. And I, tired of games, asked, "And that pleases you? After he just saved your life!"

She laughed, "You're kidding!" Then, angrily, "And over-dramatizing!"

"I don't think so."

"Did Paul say that?"

"You know he wouldn't."

"Oh, he might say anything!"

I was in the chair by the window. I felt incredibly weary. I said, "Oh, Rachel."

Then her face collapsed. She pleaded, "Don't be angry."

I went to sit on her bed, to put my arms around her.

As a gesture of goodwill, at our urging, Rachel had seen a psychologist, a colleague of Nina's at the Ackerman Institute. She had one session with him and aborted any further ones. "I can't make four o'clock; a friend is coming from out of town." That sort of thing. I listened to it once, twice, three times—the therapist was certainly giving her a lot of rope; then I blew. It was the first open fight we had had since she had been so ill. I said that for her to sabotage any help—any possible help—was irresponsible. She answered that it wasn't any of my damn business, that she didn't need to have a damned proxy-Nina put on her, that she'd find her own psychiatrist when she was back home, in Providence. I snapped that this would suit me fine, just fine. I barely managed to refrain from adding: better today than tomorrow.

What angered me especially was the fact that the one session had been productive. Rachel had been able to talk to the therapist, to discuss her difficulty in trusting, in giving up control. But I suppose what made it impossible for her to continue to see him was, indeed, that he had been sent by Nina/Paul/us, since it was we, the failed gods, who were so much of the problem. Additionally, I guess that one session may have frightened her—a lifting of the lid. When I calmed down, I felt rotten; I had been wrong. The trouble was that I tended to forget—and so, I think, did others—that Rachel's smooth knowingness in medical and psychiatric matters, her familiarity with terms and concepts, did not constitute insights, was only cerebral. Still, the fight had cleared the air between us, and in order to make up, I bought her a huge hanging plant—just what she needed desperately; going home would require a truck.

Paul released her on December 20, after twenty-one days. Under the condition that she was to stay at the shore for a quiet week, then have a visit with him. He would not promise to let her go back to school, but he would see. "I hate it when he says, 'We'll see'!" Who could blame her? Or him?

It was an odd vacation. Of course we were happy to have Rachel at home, but also dreadfully apprehensive. I constantly caught myself monitoring her expression—was she in pain, sad, scared? Mark made me get out of the house; I must have walked more icy miles during those days than I ever hope to walk again. The weather was clear and very cold, the snow pristine, endless vistas resting the eye. During the first days Rachel did not venture out at all, but she enjoyed just being there. Music pounded through the house, and she ensconced herself with all her books on the best couch, the one overlooking the pond where the wild birds presented a constant show. Most of the pond was frozen; the remaining open spots looked like convention halls at nominating time —ducks, geese, and swans, with the sea gulls running their own committees closer to the ocean, all about as raucously as their human counterparts.

When Rachel felt better, we attempted a walk. It wasn't much that first day, barely ten minutes before the pain in her legs drove tears into her eyes and I insisted that *I* was too cold to go on. But the next day we tried it again and walked a little farther. That was the day when Rachel and I, watching Mark ahead of us, saw the ice sag under him. We screamed, but the wind carried our warning in the other direction, and suddenly Mark was in water over the tops of his boots. Before the fire later, he praised those boots which had kept his wet feet warm on the way home. I couldn't refrain from several "I told you so's"; I'd warned them that the ice wasn't strong enough yet. But unfortunately, I have become the boy who cried "Wolf." Suddenly I have too many apprehensions; no one listens anymore.

Later even my fears were calmed; the pond was frozen solid, iceboats flew back and forth under their colored sails, and we walked straight across the pond, rested and sheltered in a duck-blind for a little while, then walked back. Rachel had rosy cheeks. It was New Year's Eve; she cooked up a feast, Mark and Sam clowned for the camera wearing old cowboy hats, we drank champagne, and when we sat in front of the fire, staring, getting hypnotized by the flames, I think each of us believed that perhaps it would be a happy new year after all.

Rachel came out of her appointment with Paul as up as I'd seen her in a long time. She was going back to school. "Right now?" I asked; she was still on a daily dose of sixty milligrams of Prednisone. Yes, right now, tomorrow. She would start to reduce the Prednisone by five milligrams per week and—jubilation—Paul had put her back on a hundred milligrams of 6-mercaptopurine and on twelve Azulfidine per day. Plus four Valium and Talwin for the arthritis and the headaches caused by the Azulfidine.

I cried after I put her on the plane. Pure madness! And when Mark came home at night, I raved. I had the furious sensation that Paul was setting her up for failure. "How can she possibly work while taking that kind of sedation?" I yelled. And wasn't he really indulging her in a very cynical manner, saying, in fact, "You insist on going back to school? Okay, go. It's not my concern that you'll fall asleep every time you sit down." It reminded me, I said to Mark, of something very mean I used to do to the kids when they were little and when I was at the end of my tether at the low point of the day. I'd magnanimously give them choices: "Now, look," I'd say with a sweet smile, "you can either go to bed now or in five minutes!" Poor little dopes, yelling triumphantly, "In five minutes." They didn't know they had been had. Wasn't that exactly what Paul was doing to Rachel? And why didn't she see it? And how could she be happy to be back on the immunosuppressive agent when it was she who initiated all the talk of its dangers? On and on I went.

Mark heard me out. Then he asked quietly what the alternatives were. "Think," he said. "What options did Paul have?" And wasn't it true that Rachel would have fought him tooth and nail if he'd forced her to stay home? And wouldn't the tension this would have created have aggravated her condition as well? And/or might she not have disregarded his advice anyhow and done whatever she pleased?

I had to agree with all that; but, I argued, if he had to let her go, wasn't he absolutely manufacturing terrible frustration if he sedated her to a point at which she couldn't fulfill her obligations? "I'd think the frustration would be as harmful as the tension!" And anyhow, how did we know? Perhaps if Paul had given her a firm no, she would have accepted it. Or even welcomed it.

Mark shrugged. "I doubt it. I don't think he could have stopped her. I think he took a calculated risk that the medication would slow her down at least, that the steroids and the six-MP will work, that she'll get through this attack."

"And then what?" But the anger at Paul had dissipated. If anything, I felt resentful of Rachel, then ashamed and guilty. That was all she needed on top of trying to deal with the illness and getting on with her life: her mother's annoyance because she caused us worry!

"Look," Mark was saying, "stop beating yourself. Of course we're angry. It makes as much and as little sense as her fury at us. Dear, sweet God, what's a semester? If she'd just listen . . ." He stopped, then added in a tight voice, "Anyhow, it will resolve itself."

Looking at him, I saw deep lines around his eyes. God, I suddenly thought, look at us, we are no longer young. I asked, "What do you mean, it will resolve itself?"

"It won't work. Not while she starves herself on top of it."

Now fear rose up and engulfed me, my head flushed, my chest was tight. I jumped up, frantic to change the subject; oh, I wouldn't think of it. I simply wouldn't think of it anymore. I'd take a deep breath. . . .

Thank God for closets. But at midnight when I was still half buried under a pile of clothes about which I couldn't decide— rummage or might I yet wear that old suit?—Mark said angrily to please get the junk off his bed; he was going to sleep. I then transferred my activities to Rachel's closet, and at two it was a wonder of neatness, her sweaters piled up in precise stacks, her shoes like soldiers; I would just fall into bed now and sleep.

But after a couple of hours I woke with a start and it was all back. How I hated to have her back on the 6-MP, and God, I knew just what would happen; I'd been wrong to think that the four Valium would stop her. Oh, no, she'd double her efforts and overcome their effect; she'd tax her system extra hard. And what Mark had said . . . about her not eating. She had promised me, but could she? It was ironic . . . now, after all these years, Paul was suddenly at her, talking nutrition. Oh, and why was she not mooning in spite of all the steroids? How mixed up was her body chemistry by now? And dear God, what if she'd suddenly get that pain again, the megacolon . . . in this snow, how to get her home or to a hospital? Oh, why had Paul let her go?

Suddenly, startling me, Mark said, "Come over here; let me hold you." His voice sounded absolutely awake.

"I thought you were sleeping."

He laughed; we snuggled together. "Anyhow," I said into his shoulder, "it wasn't such a crazy assumption; some people sleep at night."

In the morning as I walked around the house with a hole in my stomach, my thoughts suddenly clarified. The panic of the night was less about Rachel, perhaps, than about us. Seeing that Mark looked so worn, so . . . the word that came to me was: slashed. Oh, oh, I'd never forgive her if something happened to him. Then I stood, appalled. Until, at last, I could shake my thoughts. "I must stop this," I said out loud.

Of course, after a few days I adjusted. I was rather good at that. It was a matter of getting busy, practicing some censorship, but allowing enough steam to escape to keep from blowing up. I had experience. Anyhow, Rachel sounded okay on the telephone, even though I wasn't entirely sure that she was telling me the truth. It was "I'm fine, honest!" and "I'm telling you, I'm doing all right." But the thing that reassured me most was that she was seeing a lot of the Bradshaws and the Trumans. I had a feeling that they were keeping an eye on her. And Lenny too. "He comes every day!" Rachel said in a tone that was supposed to express exasperation. So there seemed to be no reason not to get back into my own life. I was sketching out a new novel, a college novel, perhaps set at Harvard (neutral ground).

At night I was tired and exhilarated the way I feel when I write. Which was why, when Rachel called and said, "Mom?" my heart didn't plummet; anyhow, the last three days she had said that she was really coming out of it, feeling super. "Hi, sweetheart," I answered. I was in bed already; it was eleven o'clock.

"I think I'll be on that flight that gets in around noon, Mom. The Allegheny one. Can you get me?"

Déja vù. "What's the matter?" She had spoken as through clenched teeth.

"I have this pain. Paul said to have someone give me a shot of Demerol; Douglas is on his way over."

I waited, unable to say anything, the ice traveling through me, the familiar ice.

"Mom?"

"I'm here, darling."

"I want to hang up; I'll call you later." I heard two clicks, realized that Mark had also been on, must have picked up the phone in his study. He was coming up the stairs. Then sat down heavily on the side of the bed. "So," he said.

Perhaps because we had been through moments of intense fear so often, there was a routine, almost a ritual. I talked, Mark listened. I talked calmly, sensibly, putting the situation into perspective. Then we sat and thought. Or tried—past the panic and, I realized, the fury. Then panic again: it was sleeting outside. Yesterday Rachel had said that Providence was pure ice. . . . What if Dr. Bradshaw had an accident, couldn't get to her?

Mark was reaching for the telephone. "I'm going to fly up there."

"You won't get a flight before morning."

"Then I'll drive."

"No!" I yelled; something would happen to him too. Then, a little calmer, "No, let's wait awhile, then talk to Dr. Bradshaw." We decided to give it an hour before calling back. But before the hour was up, Lenny called. He had just helped Dr. and Mrs. Bradshaw get Rachel into their car; they were taking her to Miriam Hospital. Dr. Bradshaw wanted x-rays and blood tests; he had told Len to call us and tell us that he'd be in touch after he knew a little more. Yes, Rachel was in bad pain, but he thought the Demerol had begun to work when they left; she had been dopey.

Dr. Bradshaw called at two o'clock. A nice voice. Quickly, he said that the x-rays did not indicate danger of megacolon or rupture. However, her white count was up and she was running a fever and had this pain. He had called in a gastroenterologist; they thought it might be best to get her home to her own physician. But they'd make the final decision, whether it was safe to move her, in the morning. She was comfortable now; they had given her morphine. They were keeping her in the emergency ward overnight.

Mark said he'd take the first flight in the morning and fetch her.

Dr. Bradshaw thought perhaps that would only delay matters "... in this weather!" he said. And "How about if my wife, Olivia, takes her home? Livvy is a nurse." He turned away our expressions of gratitude, he was warm, reassuring; he would talk to us in the morning.

At eight A.M. the Providence gastroenterologist called and said that together with two other colleagues he had just seen Rachel; they thought it would be all right to fly her home. The hospital social worker was making the arrangements; Mrs. Bradshaw would accompany her.

It was brilliant that day, sunny and cold. The roads were clear—snowbanks on the sides, but free of ice. I stayed in the car; Mark negotiated for the wheelchair to meet the plane at the ramp. And then there they were, Rachel giving me a sleepy crooked grin, looking like a little girl in the blue lambskin jacket I had bought for her in Milan when she was fifteen. I noted that hat and gloves did not match—very un-Rachel; it gave me a glimpse of the haste in which the Bradshaws had gotten her together in the night. Very naturally, I embraced Olivia Bradshaw; she hugged me back; we were immediate friends. In fact, this instant friendship complicated things all that day, through the fear, the hurry, the confusion, at Paul's office, in the hospital, until Mark took her back to the airport to catch a plane home in the evening, everywhere we tried to snatch a few minutes of talk. Lives to catch up on, so much to tell each other. And Rachel, through all the haze and pain, "Do you like her, Mom? Isn't she super?" Somehow, it was very important to her at that scary moment that her mother and her friend like each other.

In Paul's waiting room while he examined Rachel. Again. "I feel that I have spent half my life here," I said to Olivia, Livvie already, and she understood. But Mark too. He is usually stiff, even pompous, with strangers, but he wasn't with Livvie; we talked. Then Paul joined us. Rachel was sleeping in the x-ray room. "She has pancreatitis," he said calmly, in charge, easing the panic. "It's rare, but there are cases on record where the six-mercaptopurine has caused it." He had a bed at Lenox Hill Hospital in the intensive-care unit. "The only bed in the whole hospital," he said.

And I, sharply, "Please talk straight. Are you putting Rachel into intensive care because she is that sick or because there is no other bed?"

He answered, also with an edge in his voice, "Why would I lie? There's no other bed."

I didn't believe him.

To confirm the diagnosis of pancreatitis, the conclusive test is one that measures the quantity of certain enzymes (amylase and lipase) circulating in the blood. Of the first three tests—the one from Miriam Hospital in Providence, the one Paul took in his office, and the one made in the intensive-care unit—the first two were positive, the third not. Rachel was put on intravenous feeding to rest her pancreas, the ingestion of the 6-mercaptopurine was stopped, and within twenty-four hours she was moved out of the I.C.U. into a semiprivate room on the seventh floor. This was Paul country; his patients got a lot of care; he was respected and perhaps a little feared. I had the impression that neither nurses nor interns wanted to be recipients of one of his caustic remarks.

For Rachel this was her first experience being in the care of young doctors who worked under the supervision of an attending physician. A flock of them took her history that first day. Rachel's bed was the one nearer the door; an old lady in pink quilted robe and high blood pressure was at the window. Drawing the curtain and pretending that it was a wall offering privacy, the young doctors listened to Rachel's litany—a precise story, correct generic name of each medication, dosage, combination. I was standing in the doorway and therefore heard a pale, long-haired boy say, "Ugh, a damn pharmacist!" Then, as in contempt, he turned and walked away. I felt stunned by the heartlessness of the remark, yet wondered how Rachel had annoyed him. Was there something officious in her manner, something aggressive; had she said to him that she knew as much as he did? Yes, perhaps. Maybe it was a situation that might amuse an older doctor but was offensive to one of these youngsters with sea legs still unsteady. Fortunately, we never saw that young man again.

The two interns taking care of Rachel turned out to be terrific; Rachel liked and respected them as she did the resident, a blond young woman. I noted that the resident remained Dr. Carlsbad throughout, though the interns were soon Michael and Eddie, arguing medicine with her. One morning I heard Michael say, "Well, you were wrong and so is Dr. Zalinger; it can't be pancreatitis. I read up on it; it's not caused by six-mercaptopurine." Rachel replied heatedly that it wasn't written up *yet*. "Not yet, because Dr. Zalinger hasn't published the article yet! You'll read it soon enough!" However, the greater familiarity did not lead to contempt—it was merely a matter of style on the part of the doctors.

In the midst of the tests and x-rays of the first days, Paul suggested consulting another doctor. We were relieved that the approach came from him; the friendship was once again cutting with double edge—how could we ask for another opinion? But once the subject was broached, Mark suggested, and Paul agreed, that he consult Paul's peer at the Foundation, Dr. Aaron Ashbrook from Boston. However, the timing didn't work out and Dr. Ashbrook could not come to New York at that moment, so we only had a long talk with him on the telephone.

It became obvious to Mark and me, who were each on an extension, that on hearing Rachel's history, with special emphasis on the eleven years of *active* ulcerative colitis, Dr. Ashbrook was inclined toward recommending surgery. He used a phrase that stuck in our minds. He said that he was not of the school that would advocate surgery automatically after ten years for fear of malignancy. Rather, he said, he measured "activity times duration" in forming his opinion. He was unfavorably impressed by the fact that Rachel had not enjoyed any spontaneous remissions and not even a chemically induced one in recent years. He also spoke of the "quality of life" aspect of the situation, and he told us about a young patient, a medical student, who had recently opted for the surgery because he could no longer tolerate the life of a semi-invalid. Of course, Dr. Ashbrook made no recommendations, since he had neither seen the x-rays nor met Rachel, but we decided to stay in touch; he would try to see Rachel in a couple of weeks.

The conversation left Mark and me somehow reassured. Why? It was something in his attitude—the acceptance that medical management can fail and not represent tragedy. I said to Mark, "It's ridiculous that we need a stranger to bring us that message. All we have to do is look at Sam."

"But Paul—"

I interrupted. "Perhaps we are too concerned with not failing Paul," I said. Then stopped, appalled. I had blurted it out. Where had it come from? Could it be true? I shook my head; true or not, it was only one of many things to be considered. And it was academic. Rachel had to make the decision, not we. And she still spoke of the surgery as "out of the question," even though I had the impression again and again that she was going through a process of reevaluation.

On Paul's recommendation, we consulted the head of the department of gastroenterology at Lenox Hill, Dr. Frederick Hofman. One morning he spent a long time with Rachel, then saw us in the late afternoon at his office. I had an immediate sense of confidence, and both Mark and I admitted to each other later that he reminded us of Gustl—the soft voice, slight build, the gentleness. Perhaps most impressive, the quick insight into Rachel's character, and the weight he was giving to her personality traits as they related to the disease. He spoke of her determination, her quest to live fully, her remarkable strength. Regretfully, he said, her history, the x-ray findings, and his clinical observations obliged him to recommend the surgery. However, he was certain that she would adjust very well.

Again, leaving his office, and contrary to what one might expect, we felt comforted. "Perhaps," Mark suggested, "we have lived with the fear of cancer for so long that the surgery is the lesser evil." I nodded, yes, yes; the weird thing was only how deep we had kept this fear hidden. Deep enough for us to manage to live.

I had promised Rachel that we'd stop by at the hospital and tell her about the consultation. We found her sitting up in bed, the curtain drawn between her and a new neighbor, two red spots—like clown makeup—high on her cheekbones. She was outraged. And like a sudden cloudburst, a torrent of abuse, mainly directed at Mark: how could he have done this to her? How could he have a consultation behind her back as if she were a child? No, one oughtn't even do that to a child! And didn't Mark understand that he was violating her most sacred convictions?—the right of the patient to know, to be part of the process of evaluation.

We stood there, thoroughly scolded. Mark, at least, was completely surprised. I, however, thought ruefully that I might have prevented the outburst if I had been more sensitive. Rachel had complained to me earlier—how could we have this consultation without her? I argued that it would make Mark nervous to speak in front of her, had said jokingly, "You know Daddy with his million questions; you'd inhibit him." Then, when Paul had happened by, he had said easily, "Oh Rachel, let your father have this talk for *his* peace of mind." Rachel said no more, and I thought that we had convinced her. But no. As she waited for us, the indignation had grown mightily.

It took a while to calm her. Mark defended his view, said that after all, she had complete and constant access to Dr. Hofman, she could ask him anything, have her own consultation; why wasn't he entitled, why didn't he have the right, to also get information in a manner conducive to his psychic needs?

At that Rachel's indignation flared anew. "Because it's *I* who's sick!" she whispered fiercely. The lady behind the curtain was very sick; her oxygen tank hissed constantly; her cough wrung my heart. Pointing a finger at Mark, Rachel added, "What would you do if I were married? Would you also have the 'right'?"

"I'd think your husband would grant it to me."

"But you wouldn't *take* it for granted. No, it's because you pay the bills that you think you can—"

"Rachel!" I interjected.

But Mark was saying stiffly that he was sorry; he hadn't realized that she was feeling that strongly.

"You ought to. Don't you ever listen to me? Don't you hear what I say, what I am?" Then, with tears of reproach in her eyes, "Mom could have told you."

I too apologized. But inside, I was angry. She was being damned ungenerous. She didn't take Mark's need into consideration at all or give a hoot that this was hard on us too. But later, after some thought, and as we were driving home, I answered myself. "She can't afford to be generous right now," I said to Mark. "She's got too much on her plate."

"I know," he replied.

The next morning I walked into another crisis. Rachel was again beside herself. I tried a small joke before I realized the seriousness. "Once more?" I asked. "We're going to fight once more?"

"It isn't funny. Everyone is lying to me. Paul, you . . ."

"Hey, whoa. . . ." I took her hands; they were moist and hot; her eyes were dilated. Serious at last, I asked, "What happened?"

Paul had been in early that morning. She had asked him what Dr. Hofman had said, and he had replied that he had not yet consulted with him, that he would see him later, that he didn't know what Dr. Hofman's evaluation had been. As for us, we had certainly been evasive last night.

I interrupted. "That isn't fair, Rachel. In fact, if you recall, we were only discussing the question of the right or wrong of our having seen Dr. Hofman without you. You were so disturbed that

226

we didn't even get around to talking about the content of the consultation. But you know I am going to tell you everything; that's why I'm here."

"Well, you're too late." Michael had been in that morning on his rounds, together with a few other interns. They had been very nice to her, had sat down, asked her how she felt about Dr. Hofman's suggestion. "I tried to pretend that I knew what they were talking about, but Michael noticed that I was faking. He felt bad, but then he told me that it said in the chart that Dr. Hofman recommended the surgery; he was sure that I knew."

"I'm sorry that you heard it like that," I said, "but it's a question of a half hour, isn't it? No one was trying to keep it from you."

"Paul was."

"I don't know. Perhaps he didn't have the time to go into it at that moment. Or perhaps he wanted to speak to Dr. Hofman more thoroughly before he made comment; he'd hardly want to discuss a mere note in a chart with you." Just then I saw that Rachel was looking at someone over my shoulder. I turned, and there was Paul. "Oh, I am glad you're here," I called out, and explained.

Refusing my offer of the chair, Paul leaned against the wall. He looked tired. I tried to push against the wave of sympathy for him that rose in me. No, I could not be concerned with what this was doing to him, whether it represented failure; I had to worry about evaluating it, checking it against reality. . . .

"What is it you want to know, Rachel?" he was asking. "I've just had a talk with Dr. Hofman; he will be in shortly to see you."

"I want to know why he—no, never mind; I'll ask him that myself. I want to know whether you agree with him, whether you've changed your mind that I'm not a candidate for the surgery."

We watched Paul's face. It was all there, the concentration, the honesty. He said, "No. No, I have not changed my mind. At this moment, I do not consider you—"

She interrupted. "What does that mean: at this moment?"

"Just what it says, Rachel."

"In other words: tomorrow you might feel different?"

"I don't know."

"All right, let me ask you this: what could change your mind?"

"There could arise clinical circumstances that would make me have to opt for the surgery."

"But waiting for them—doesn't that diminish your chance to choose *elective* surgery?"

"Perhaps. It's a matter of judgment."

"I see."

They were staring at each other. Then Paul turned to me. "Jean?" he asked.

I shook my head. Rachel had asked the pertinent questions.

"All right, then let me go see my sick patients!" And in the door, "Your white count is normal today."

He was hardly out of earshot when she wailed, "He didn't say that, did he? Would you believe it?" Then we burst into laughter. Dr. Hofman walked into it, looked surprised, then pleased. But it seemed too much effort to explain the joke. Outside, I wondered whether I should have stayed. Did Rachel want her "equal time," or had she wanted me there? Then realized that it didn't matter. I recalled her look of concentration, her face full of tension; Dr. Hofman had sat down on the side of the bed, had taken her hand.

He was with her for almost an hour, and when he came out he stopped to tell me again what a remarkable girl Rachel was. I wanted to ask question after question, especially the one that occurred to me during the night—was there any specific thing in the x-ray, other than active ulcerative colitis, that made him recommend surgery? Was there some area that indicated a possible malignancy? But he was patting my arm, and I felt that he was anxious to be off. No, I mustn't dance around and around; I'd have to cope with these thoughts on my own. I apologized for delaying him, but he said nonsense, anything, anytime at all.

Rachel wanted to know what he had said in the hall; I repeated it almost verbatim. She nodded, said, "Yes, Dr. Grossman is also in favor of the surgery."

"Steven? When did you speak to him?"

"He comes by every morning; he's explained all about the Kock procedure. He's really nice."

"Wait a minute—"

"You know, the continent ileostomy."

"Yes, I've heard of it, but I know nothing about it." No, nothing; I'd been pushing it out of my mind again and again. But Rachel had informed herself.

She was saying, "Paul has said to me that if he were ever to have to consider surgery, he would only recommend the Kock for me. I think we should all have a consultation with Dr. Grossman to find out more."

"All right," I replied, shell-shocked. Things were going too fast. Or perhaps not. Because now Rachel was saying, "Of course, it's not acute. Paul says . . ." Then she stopped and thought. "But Dr. Grossman says that the Kock procedure cannot be performed under emergency conditions, that it has to be done electively, practically in an ideal situation. He doesn't recommend it."

"I thought you said he does."

"No. He recommends surgery, but not the Kock procedure."

"And Paul does not recommend surgery, but yes, the—what's it called?"

"The name is continent, or reservoir, ileostomy. But since it was invented by this doctor named Kock in Sweden, they call it that too. With a 'K.' " Suddenly she grabbed my hand. "Everyone says something different, Mom."

"I know. It scares me."

"If the white count is normal, maybe I'm coming out of it."

"Are you still bleeding?"

"But not so bad. It's the headaches and my legs that are the worst."

"That could be from the steroids and the Azulfidine."

"I know. I don't even know which is which anymore. Those damn drugs."

The lady behind the curtain was coughing badly. I had never seen her; the curtain was always closed. Sometimes Rachel and I smiled as we listened to one of her visitors reading poetry to her over there in the window world; it seemed both strange and nice. Rachel called, "Are you all right, Julie?"

A hoarse voice answered, "Yes."

"Shall I ring for the nurse?"

"No, I can reach my bell. Thanks, Rachel."

I felt surprised; I hadn't known that Rachel had any contact with her. Rachel answered my unspoken question: "We talk at night. She's got kids my age."

A little later, Rachel got one of the terrible headaches which really took her out of commission. Leaving her to sleep it off, I sat downstairs in the cafeteria and stared into my tea. But she is better, I argued. Better than the day she had come to the hospital, better than I had seen her many times. Her white count was normal. And the intravenous feeding had been stopped; Rachel was eating soft foods—well, mostly D-Zerta and sherbet—without stomach pains. And now the headaches. But anyone would have a headache after such a morning; I had one. This talking, over and under. Or had I already made up my mind? Even if it was not for me to decide. Oh, God, I had to be so careful not to influence Rachel. But how was she to make a decision; who'd have the courage? And if she couldn't, if an emergency forced action on her? Then she wouldn't be able to have the new operation. Yes, I must find out about it; it was time, it was high time that I inform myself.

CHAPTER 13

FROM RACHEL'S POEM:
AT LAST, THE FOREST A CATHEDRAL

The new God, the old one failed, you know.
Just a man, a doctor.
A new chance, a better way.
Orderly,
trees planted in a row.

I was still in the dream; Rachel was screaming. I was trying to determine whether it was fury or pain that caused the sound in my ear. But suddenly knew that I was awake, was listening intently on the telephone. I groped for the bedside clock, looked through slitted eyes—yes, it was eight thirty; I had overslept. "Start again, Rachel," I begged. "I'm groggy from a pill I took at three."

"The son of a bitch! Without consulting me. Just marched in— both of them, Michael and Eddie—and said that Paul had ordered it." They had reestablished the intravenous, had restarted the high steroids."

"But why, Rachel, why?"

"Because of the pain. And I'm running a hundred and three."

I was coming awake. The reason I had not slept until so late was the hour we had spent on the telephone with Paul the previous night. We had pressed him, I realized with a start. We had said, Do something, in all kinds of ways. Our questions had solidified into a kind of attack. We wanted answers; no, we wanted assurances. "Look, assuming that the disease enters a state of remission," Mark had insisted, "is there a chance that the affected section of the colon can recover its functional utility? Can it regenerate itself?" And I had wanted to know why he was so much less scared of malignancy than everyone else. Mark had interrupted me before I could count off their names—Dr. Ashbrook, Dr. Hofman, Dr. Bradshaw, Dr. Grossman—so I had switched to my other obsession and asked what, if there should be no remission, were the risks of continued infusion of heavy dosages of steroids and immunosuppressive agents and Azulfidine and . . . "Yes, and how about the secondary effects such as relate to childbearing?"

Paul had answered patiently, honestly. Several times he had said he didn't have the answer to that. At some point it had become clear to me that he was saying that it was a matter of intangibles, his judgment versus the platitudes, his evaluation of the situation from day to day against generalities—it was a matter of trust. Oh, God, I had thought in the hours during which I had tossed sleeplessly, how much trust is sane?

Now I felt panicked with guilt about these thoughts. Did they push Paul into shooting off big guns in this autocratic manner? Oh, swept by guilt—we had nagged and niggled; Paul was tired of the combined Bergman clan arguing, arguing. . . .

I said, "Rachel, he must have a reason. Wait till he gets there."

But she was not to be calmed. Voice high, "He better be here quick, because I'm going to rip this damn needle out of my arm right now, and I'm going to sign myself out of here before you can bat an eye."

"Rachel, listen . . ."

"I can't think of one single reason in the world why this couldn't have waited until he got here and explained it to me."

Now I was yelling too. "Stop it! For God's sake, what the hell difference does it make? The important thing seems to be that he wanted the medication in you quickly. What is it, steroids and an antibiotic?"

"No, just ACTH." And the rising voice again. "And I don't want any more, I don't want any more." She was sobbing.

I tried speaking in a very quiet tone. At last she seemed to be listening. I would be there in thirty minutes; hold on, just hold on. I laid the telephone down on her weeping.

But when I got there, it was the same. Except no more tears, just determination. She wanted the I.V. out; this minute she wanted it out. And she wanted no more steroids; it was time to unmask the situation, to find out what was making her ill, the disease or the drugs.

I argued. "You may be doing something dangerous, it isn't up to you to make such decisions, you may be precipitating an emergency, you know one cannot stop steroids abruptly—"

"You can when it's only an hour since they were started." She looked up at the bottle, the inexorable drip, drip. Then cried out, "Mom, please. No more; I cannot stand any more of that stuff in me."

All the time I was holding her hands, fighting the panic in myself, agreeing with her on all kinds of levels, but thinking that I must not, I must not abet her hysteria, must not be drawn into it.

Then Paul was there. Calm, quietly spoken. "What is it you want, Rachel?"

"I want this out." She held out her arm.

"All right." Deliberately, he stepped closer, peeled off the adhesive that was holding the I.V. to the arm, tore open a silver-foiled alcohol swab, pulled out the needle, and applied pressure to the little wound. "There," he said. "Now can we talk?"

Quickly, I left the room. Mark had also arrived in the meantime; I filled him in, and over and over we replayed the scene. We were both wondering whether Rachel might be having some kind of psychotic episode. To rebel against the doctor. To insist the I.V. be taken out. To say that she refused to be dosed with more steroids. Yet all of it made a type of sense; none of it was "crazy," not under the circumstances. Then Paul came to join us, and to my tremendous relief, he agreed. No, it was not crazy; it was as good a way as any to proceed, if that was how she felt about it. "Let's unmask the situation," he said, using her phrase. He put his arm around me, acknowledging without words the hard time we were sharing. Yet none of us said it—it might be fine, good, the way to go about it. Or it might end up in surgery by nighttime. "What is the fever, the pain?" I asked.

"I don't really know."

"Could it be some leakage into the abdominal cavity?"

It could be; we would have to sit tight. The important thing right now was to keep Rachel calm; don't have her blow it! And all three of us smiled at the *double entendre*. I thought, it is we who are mad, making jokes about the danger of rupture.

It was Saturday, but Dr. Hofman looked in and Dr. Grossman

was very much around. But finally everyone went off. Rachel was calm and very tired. I told Mark to keep his business appointment as planned, got myself a cup of coffee and a sandwich, and sat quietly with Rachel. I had finally met her neighbor, had apologized to her for the commotion of the morning. "Don't be silly," she had said, "God, the poor kid!" I thought that she was a pretty poor kid herself—she had emphysema—but she was terrific, just as Rachel had said. Now the curtain was closed again; Julie's oxygen hissed; after the turmoil of the morning it was almost cozy, a respite. Rachel lay rubbing the area where the I.V. had left a bruise. "If I could only talk to Adam Truman," she mused.

"Dr. Truman couldn't be your psychologist anyhow. He's your friend."

"I know. I mean just to talk. And he'd find someone . . ." I saw that the premise was still the return to Providence. But I nodded, began to play with the thought of calling him; might he come?

The nurse who had taken Rachel's temperature a few minutes earlier was back and stuck the thermometer into Rachel's mouth again. I asked, "Hey, didn't you just do that a little while ago?"

"Just checking," she said. Lenox Hill was using the newfangled electric thermometers; the whole procedure took only a minute. A moment later she was there again, this time with a blood-pressure cuff. And then Eddie came. Eddie had red hair. Ordinarily one didn't notice his freckles, but they stood out sharply in his pale face just then. He asked Rachel how she felt, he took her pulse, he watched her and shook his head. Then he left. I followed him outside. "Is anything the matter?" I asked.

"She's running a bit of a temperature," he answered, and sped off.

I followed him down the hall slowly; panic was gathering again. Now what? I was walking carefully—not sneaking up to the desk, or hiding myself or anything like that, but I certainly tried to be unobtrusive. And so I saw Eddie talking into the phone, gesticulating with his other hand, and I heard the nurses talk about the fact that Racel had a hundred five. Which is when it grabbed me, a giant hand in my guts; I ran, I sped down that corridor; fortunately, the toilet was unoccupied. My insides were spilling out in waves.

By the time I could walk again, soaked, my blouse sticking to me, I was shivering and weak but determined. I stopped at the desk, I told them to call Dr. Zalinger immediately. The nurse smiled at me, Eddie too—it was a mistake, they said. They had called Dr. Zalinger, all right; he had told them to get a different thermometer. The new one had registered a reasonable hundred and two. "Boy, I was scared," the nurse said, too relieved to be embarrassed. Me too, I owned.

By evening it made a funny story. Guess what happened this afternoon after all that happened this morning? We stood in front of Rachel's room, Nina and Paul and some of our friends. Sam was with Rachel; she just wanted Sam. "How did you know that it was a broken thermometer?" I asked Paul. "After all, for her fever to shoot up was exactly what we were afraid of."

"But not that quickly. I had just seen her an hour earlier," he answered.

At last we went off for dinner, leaving Sam with Rachel. Kissing her good night, I told her that Dr. Truman would be with her the next day. Mark had called him, told him the situation, asked whether he'd make a professional call. He said that he would come, of course. "But not professionally! Rachel's our friend. I'll take an early train."

Rachel cried.

"You've got some friends!" I said, thinking, as I had often thought, about this quality in Rachel that led to these extraordinary relationships.

"And his wife is just as dear," she assured me.

At dinner, with the conversation swirling around me, with the drink hitting powerfully into my emptiness, the day didn't seem possible.

Adam Truman sat at Rachel's bedside for six hours. Then Mark took him to Penn Station to catch his train back to Providence. Of course, we didn't know what it was that they had said, but Rachel was calmer. And yet perhaps more determined. She would not go back on steroids. But she would see a psychiatrist to help her make up her mind. And she wanted to explore the idea of the surgery. "Let's have that consultation with Dr. Grossman," she decreed.

The strange thing was that Rachel showed an initial improvement once she was off the steroids. The state of alarm during which we stood by, prepared for—if not actually expecting—disaster, passed; we realized that we had a respite during which we could explore the question of whether and which surgery would be necessary; we could make up our minds calmly. However, none of us ever recovered a sufficiently peaceful state of mind to do anything except proceed forthwith. The interview with Dr. Grossman was scheduled for Monday, and on Tuesday we would meet with a psychiatrist who had served as consultant and referrer to us since we'd had our very first problem some thirty years earlier just before we got married.

The consultation with Dr. Grossman was held under the new ground rules—together with Rachel. For Mark this was a terrible ordeal, and it certainly added to my anxiety as well. I was not at all sure that Mark would be able to accept Rachel's condition, and I half feared that he'd be uncooperative in an unconscious kind of passive resistance. Anticipating such a situation and the resultant pressure it would place on me, I swung madly between anger at Mark's inflexibility and anger at Rachel's intransigence. However, I need not have worried. Mark was able to overcome his inhibitions, and between Rachel, him, and me, I think we managed to ask every question that was on our minds. First, though, we listened to Dr. Grossman recommend surgery—a reasoned, calm presentation which contained the elements we were already familiar with as well as the statement that since the surgery was not permanently avoidable, it was very desirable to schedule it for a moment of relative calm, as early as possible. Yes, he too felt that the ten-plus years of active illness lent weight to a legitimate worry about malignancy.

At first I felt impatient while he spoke, anxious to have him proceed to a discussion of the new operation; but he was not to be hurried. There was logic in the way he built his case, there was a reassuring quality that was cumulative—he was obviously more than just a "knife man"—and I began to relax. Which made it harder to discount the obviously negative presentation he gave to the continent ileostomy.

After explaining that the operation involved the construction of a reservoir and a nipple valve fashioned out of approximately forty cm. of the end of the ileum, of which ten are used for the valve and outflow and the remaining thirty for the pouch, and that this procedure is done in conjunction with a total proctocolectomy, he said that the length of the surgery is approximately six to seven hours, that very extensive internal suturing is involved, and that these factors increase the risk of the operation considerably.

He appeared also to have reservations about its alleged improvement in life-style, since he felt that the dangers of even an established continent ileostomy were likely to restrict the patient to the vicinity of surgical assistance at all times, and that the procedure rendered the patient more dependent than someone who had a conventional ileostomy.

He stressed the uncomplicated life of the person who wears an appliance outside the body; he emphasized that the operation for this kind of ileostomy had been perfected to a point at which he and his associate performed it in less than two hours, and he told us that several medical centers in the United States had abandoned doing the Kock procedure because of poor results. Listening, I became more and more bewildered that he appeared to be willing to perform the operation at all. However, he said that he would do so "if Rachel insisted on it."

We brought up the point that the operation was being performed successfully at Mt. Sinai Hospital by Dr. Gaon, and Dr. Grossman owned that yes, so he had heard, but so far there was very little published information available.

Afterward, we mulled it over: his saying that he was a conservative man who would choose the procedure neither for himself nor for his daughter; his declaring that the extensive sutures on the inside of the body, "once the incision has been closed, are left to the mercy of God"; and his warning about the problems that could arise when intubation did not work properly. "Well," Mark said, "Either he's one of those people who have to cover their backs for every possibility, or he was giving us a message!"

"A message!" I said. "Loud and clear: don't!"

We had returned to Rachel's room after consulting in an office at the other end of the corridor. Rachel was exhausted from the trek, lay very pale, listening to us. "I can't quite understand why Paul recommends this procedure if it's as dangerous as Dr. Grossman says," I said. "Perhaps we should forget about it."

"Then you can forget about surgery: period." Rachel intervened. "You might as well know, the continent ileostomy is the only one I'll consider." Her face had flushed.

We studied the diagram Dr. Grossman had drawn for us. The pouch in which waste collected would be situated in the cavity created by the removal of the colon; it would lie behind the bladder, and its neck, or outflow, would stretch into an outlet in the right lower quadrant of the abdomen, approximately between the pelvic bone and the pubic symphysis. This stoma would be closed by an inverted nipple valve, which was the instrument of the reservoir's continence. To intubate, a plastic catheter would be inserted into this valve. Intubation was necessary two to three times per day. "An incredible piece of engineering," I marveled.

"If it works," Mark said.

"It works marvelously. Paul said so," Rachel insisted.

Paul had suggested—in case the surgery was decided upon—that Dr. Gaon would join Dr. Grossman in performing the operation. This seemed to us an unrealistic plan, and Dr. Grossman, when we had mentioned it, had seemed less than enthusiastic. And why should Gaon operate at Lenox Hill when he was affiliated with Mt. Sinai? Suddenly the whole thing seemed murky, impossible. "I think a consultation with Dr. Gaon is in order," I suggested.

We agreed to ask Paul to arrange it.

Exhausted, discouraged, Mark and I kicked it back and forth on our way home. The trouble was that we liked Dr. Grossman, that Paul had sold us on his brilliance, that his thoughtful and thorough presentation had made an awful lot of sense. Now suddenly there was the new problem—the rather clear indication that if Rachel insisted on this particular operation, Dr. Grossman was probably the wrong surgeon. And who could blame Rachel for wanting to reach for it? The cosmetic advantages were staggering. And perhaps the psychological ones as well. "Don't you understand?" she had said just before we left. "Don't you see how much easier it would be for me? The quality of life . . ." she had stopped; tears had gathered in her eyes.

"We'll talk about it tomorrow," I had said, hoping to soothe her.

Mark mused, "I don't see how the quality of life will be better if she's got to stick close to a good hospital all the time. You know how Rachel chafes under restrictions."

"But he said that this would only be the case for a while, a year or so. Then she can go wherever she wants."

"Did Steven Grossman say that?"

"No. But Rachel said that Paul had said so." I added angrily, "For someone who's against the operation *per se*, he has certainly put a bee in Rachel's bonnet."

When we got home, we called him. He was amazed at the negative stand *vis-à-vis* the continent ileostomy Dr. Grossman had taken. Of course he'd arrange an appointment with Gaon. Then there was a pause. Perhaps all of us were thinking of the fact that if Rachel were to have the surgery at Mt. Sinai, Paul couldn't be her attending physician. He ended the silence by saying in a positive voice that the continent ileostomy was the only right choice for Rachel. "In fact, it would be the only choice I'd make for myself or the kids and Nina." Another small silence, and "However, I don't know that we have arrived at the moment . . ."

"Nothing like a little consensus!" Mark said ironically when we were going to bed. And very intensely, "Oh, God, if we're only granted the time to decide. And if Rachel can have a little while to work it through with someone."

"All this conversation presupposes that we will. If an emergency arises, the whole thing's out the window anyhow."

The next day we tried to capsule all these considerations into forty-five minutes with the psychiatrist. At the same time, working as a team, dribbling the ball back and forth, Mark and I attempted to give Dr. Goddard Rachel's history, a glimpse into her nature and character, and a rundown on her relationship with Sam, as well as the story of us as a family. We also asked him to recommend a doctor who'd see Rachel immediately and intensively. Perhaps, we suggested, he ought to be young. Certainly, he must be wise. "She needs support," I said, "I mean, over and above ours, to make these incredible decisions." And Mark agreed and added his recurring anxiety: "We just hope that she'll have the time to work this out properly."

"But if she doesn't, she'll need help even more urgently," I added.

Dr. Goddard kept nodding his head. With very few comments he made it clear that he understood the situation exactly, that he had grasped all the essentials. "It's because psychiatrists know how to really listen," Mark said to me later. "And because they don't waste half the time projecting their own egos the way other doctors do," I agreed.

"Just the same, there aren't many like Dr. Goddard!" Mark sounded a little smug. Dr. Goddard was "his" by virtue of the fact that he had counseled Mark at a moment of crisis in our youth. He said, his thoughts apparently running parallel to mine, "You know, we weren't so much older than Rachel is now."

We had parted with the understanding that Dr. Goddard would find a suitable therapist for Rachel; he would be in touch with us, perhaps as soon as that evening. But when we returned to the hospital, Rachel had just spoken to Dr. Truman. Putting the receiver down, she said, "Adam found someone for me!" He was excellently trained and connected with Einstein. Dr. Truman had spoken to him and he was willing to take Rachel's case.

"Look," I suggested, "how about letting Dr. Goddard check him out?" I was aware of the obvious advantage of someone who came recommended by Rachel's own friend, yet I was loath to give up the additional security of Dr. Goddard's approval. "Do you mind?"

"No, that's okay." And so, hardly two hours after leaving his office, Mark called Dr. Goddard back and asked him to consider the name of Benjamin Freund as well. By the following day it was all settled; Dr. Goddard had checked into the young doctor's background and found him absolutely qualified.

Thursday was the first cheerful day. There seemed no doubt that Rachel was better; the fever was down, she was even bleeding less; her gamble had not had any dire results. Now everyone spoke with respect of her "courageous" decision. She grinned at me. "From hysterical nut to wise young woman all in one easy jump!"

"Yes, but you know what everyone would have said if it had turned out differently," I came back.

"Right! Including you."

"God, I was scared."

"I know." Then she turned serious. "I realize that you thought that I was hysterical," she said. "But I really wasn't. I just had to come on so strong to make myself heard; no one would listen to me. Though inside I was really calm. In fact, I was never as sure of anything in my life as I was that I wasn't going to put more of those drugs into me."

"Just the same, it could have landed you in the O.R. Did you know that?"

"A calculated risk," she said ironically, and then seriously again, "Yes and no. I tried not to think of it."

"Still," I mused, "you must have been much more prepared for the thought of the surgery than you admitted. I know, even last summer I used to get the feeling that you were readying your mind, that you wanted me to speak of it."

"No. No, that's not true," Rachel argued. "No, I never considered it a possibility until Saturday. And *then* I felt that I was being raped." She paused, thought, added, "I still do."

We were both silent. I was censoring my thoughts, deciding that there was no advantage in pointing out that an unconscious process of taking the possibility of the surgery seriously had been in operation for a long time. And no sense whatsoever to say that I thought that she had already opted for it. That was a realization that had to come to her by her own readiness; perhaps the psychiatrist would be able to help her with that. Oh, high time for me to butt out. . . .

The other cheerful thing was Rachel's transfer that morning to a private room. Yet it had also been a wrench; she had become attached to Julie. "Such a gentle lady," she said, and bade her good-bye with tears in her eyes and promises that they'd visit each other—how many steps down the hall? My association was cynical: I thought of shipboard romances. Even though they had shared each other's most relevant crises—sure, what's more relevant than life and death? They would be forever connected. But now Rachel had a small room down the hall; we put up posters and hung flowerpots; I got her an ice bucket for her D-Zertas. She would have privacy to speak to the psychiatrist.

Dr. Benjamin Freund had fairly long hair, a beard, pink cheeks, and a shy manner. He wore a navy blue double-breasted wool trench coat and a flowing scarf. I was in love with him immediately as I scurried from the room; mothers must not intrude. Dear God, I placed a lot of reliance on him, a lot of trust and hope and expectation. He was going to help her be wise, wise beyond my own capacity. On some level, I was not unaware of how ridiculous I was. On another, I forgave myself. It was a time to believe in gods, because the need was so great.

Rachel's judgment of him was "I can talk to him!" Very fine, I supposed, even if it didn't live up to the superlatives I would have liked her to scatter forth. However, we didn't discuss it much on that day; Mark and I were going home early for a home-cooked meal because Joel and Bob and Candy and Brett, friends from school, were coming to visit Rachel. They brought Chinese food and wine and had a party in her room. Around nine the nurse came in, saw a happy Rachel, and said that she guessed they knew that visiting hours were over. Then forgot to come back. At one o'clock, Rachel's friends tiptoed out, down the silent corridor to the elevator.

Our appointment with Dr. Gaon was at his office, and Rachel had received permission to leave Lenox Hill to attend it. A nasty day; I begged Rachel to wear my coat over the skirt and shirt that were all she had at the hospital, but it had the "wrong look." I told myself to stop fussing, but somehow it was harder to acquiesce to the small foolishness than to the big issues. What if she caught a cold on top of everything?

After Dr. Gaon had examined Rachel and studied the x-rays and made his recommendation for the surgery, his presentation of the continent ileostomy did not differ very much from Dr. Grossman's. He drew the same diagrams, and he too used his index finger to illustrate the valve inside his loosely closed fist, alias the pouch. And though he had a paper titled "Continent Ileostomy in the Pediatric Patient" that had appeared in the *Journal of Pediatric Surgery* in October 1976 and which had drawings that clarified the surgical procedure some more, we realized that we were fairly well informed.

The difference was in attitude! Dr. Gaon was completely positive in his approach to the procedure, full of passionate zeal, bursting with anecdotes, speaking from experience. Later we learned the origin of his own involvement with the procedure, found out that his enthusiasm for its potential had led him to leave his practice for several months of study with Dr. Nils Kock in Göteborg, and that he had, in the meantime, improved the continence of the valve by some modification of his own. He had done more than eighty procedures; there had been no casualties.

We grilled him hard; we had plenty of ammunition: all the horrors, all the negative aspects, all the dangers about which Dr. Grossman had told us. Gaon answered readily. Nothing Dr. Grossman had said was wrong, these dangers did indeed exist, these complications could arise, the surgery was lengthy and complicated. "But," he said, "we've got answers to these problems! Answers, antidotes, precautions, remedies!"

To our question why, when so many other centers of medicine had abandoned doing this piece of surgery, he was performing it successfully, he gave an attractive small shrug. It wasn't only surgical skill, he said; there were two other matters of prime importance: selection of candidates and aftercare. Only those patients for whom the operation was clinically indicated were eligible, but unfortunately one could not really know that until one was into the surgery. For instance, he explained, "If I find an unsuspected involvement of the terminal ileum, I will not perform a continent ileostomy." Then there was the matter of selecting a patient of reliable habits, intelligence, and emotional stability, because everything depended on his or her ability to handle the crucial period of recuperation.

He outlined briefly what this involved, starting with the empty-ing of the pouch on an hourly basis, its slow progression to two-, three-, four-hour intervals, the weeks of sleep deprivation and the need for meticulous observation of his rules on how to intubate and irrigate. He also explained that immediately after the surgery the pouch was no larger than a lemon, holding only minute amounts of waste, but if correctly and slowly stretched, its capacity over several months would increase to the point at which it was able to contain between a pint and a half and one quart and attain the size of a football.

He directed most of this at Rachel; I had the feeling that he was observing her reactions carefully. At the same time, he gave Mark and me every chance to interject our questions. He was direct; he discussed the two cases that had been failures, though one of them, a case in which a very young girl had gone into a rapid growing spurt following the surgery, he felt certain he could correct once she had attained her full growth. He also pointed out to Rachel that he could not promise her to perform the procedure even though she appeared to be a candidate for it. "I know it's hard to go into this without any guarantees," he said. "For instance, if it turns out during the surgery that you're not doing well, I might decide to establish a conventional ileostomy, which cuts down the duration of the operation by several hours." He added that, in such a case, he liked to convert to the continent ileostomy about a year later. "By that time your body has had a chance to recover from the ulcerative colitis. You come into surgery as a healthy person, not debilitated as you might be at present."

Rachel nodded, apparently satisfied. Our questions were slow-ing down; I, for one, was feeling glutted. At the same time I had a fantastic sense of relief, a conviction that we were dealing with a reliable, knowing, responsible man. I recalled Paul's description of him as an all-around, complete physician, not merely a surgeon. On top of which he was charming, very warm—of course he would try to get Rachel home in time for the matzo balls; she was dimpling back; they discussed Israel and Rachel's time at Hadassah and that Dr. Gaon would teach there during the following summer. "Bring The Word to the natives," she joked. "Or anyhow, the pouch!" he agreed.

As I watched, I suddenly heard Rachel say "when," not "if," heard her discuss plans for "afterwards"; I even detected a certain tone of excitement at the challenge. And as I wondered whether she knew that she had crossed the line, that she had decided, my breath constricted; I turned cold, then very warm. And tears burned behind my eyes. Suddenly it was serious, all the speculation, all the investigation, all the talk, talk, talk. Was it my fears, perhaps, that had brought us to this point? Had I influenced Rachel, sapped her courage?

Back in her bed at Lenox Hill, she reported in minute detail to Lenny over the telephone. "No, I'll have to go to Mount Sinai for the operation. Dr. Gaon has his specially trained team of nurses and interns and residents there; it'd be silly to do it anyplace else." And "Yes, I told you, my folks have known him already since Sam had his surgery; he was the chief surgical resident then. And Dad says he's very highly regarded in the Foundation." She spoke excitedly, much louder than usual. I stood by the window, looking into the grayness outside. Eleven years of fighting. Now this. Depression like bronchitis on my chest, I struggled to breathe.

It was Sam who turned my desolation around. The eleven years had not been wasted, he said; they were enabling her to reach for the continent ileostomy, a procedure that hadn't existed in his day. He sat at the bedside and held Rachel's hand. Her face shone; Sam's approbation was like a seal. I wondered whether she understood the emotion he must be experiencing. But of course, it was nothing Sam would ever verbalize.

And now, with Rachel's conviction becoming more anchored each day, though not yet officially proclaimed, Mark's and my doubts doubled. To begin with, there was the odd phenomenon of the positive improvement in her condition. Paul spoke of letting her go home. Altogether, Paul presented a definite problem—his attitude toward the surgery was terribly ambivalent. He veered and shifted. One day he said that she was not a candidate; on another that, regrettably, it seemed that we were heading toward the surgery; and then again: "But it need not be!" in a kind of anger. And I would wonder: need not be *if?* If Rachel were not Rachel? But Rachel was Rachel.

"I don't accept the whole premise!" Rachel said angrily.

And neither did I. "More likely," I mused to Mark, "Paul just can't bear it. Either because of its taste of defeat, or because he's too involved with Rachel. And with us." But I was veering and shifting too. Next I'd defend Paul. "Poor Paul!" And I'd enumerate his troubles with the intractable Rachel.

There was now a subterranean struggle between Rachel and

Paul which took place parallel to the problems on the table. Up front was Paul's request to have her try to spend a few months resting, taking only Azulfidine and eating a nutritious diet. To this Rachel replied, "But what makes him think that I wouldn't have another exacerbation soon? I mean, I've not had a remission in years even *with* the steroids and six-MP."

And he'd say that he didn't know, but what was the harm in trying?

The harm in trying something that was useless was that it would cost her half a year and her whole research project—if we'd all kindly remember that the participants in her research were not in a position to stick around and wait for Paul to make experiments. "I really can't stand to have life postponed indefinitely," she cried, and "I can't bear any more of this half-existence." No, if she didn't opt for the surgery now, she'd go back to school.

"That's out of the question," Paul replied. "I'm sorry, but I can't permit that."

A deadlock.

So where were we to go with our doubts? Of course, there were always our friends. Our dear, dear friends for whom all this was also terribly hard. For weeks we had tried to avoid asking them for actual advice—who'd be able to bear such responsibility? Instead, we were using them as sounding boards, as lightning rods.

All except one. Mark's closest friend. Mine too. A man more completely adult than most people, a man whose opinion we both valued. And whose strength was equal to an involvement. Yes, it would ease us to know what he thought. And he was already directly involved because of his relationship with Rachel, who also trusted him. He was telephoning her daily. In fact, I didn't realize that there was that much contact until one day when she quoted him and I replied in astonishment, "But when did he say that? He's in Europe on a business trip."

"I know. He called from Amsterdam last night." She laughed. "It was some ungodly hour there."

Mark went to see him the night after he returned. And didn't come home until very, very late.

I had begun to feel frantic. "What happened?" I asked.

"I missed the turnoff into the New York Thruway. It took forever to come across the Tappan Zee Bridge."

Annoyed, I countered, "For heaven's sake, we've taken that route a million times. How could you miss it?"

"I wasn't seeing so well. I was crying."

I didn't ask what our friend had said. Not that night. To speak
of such matters at night would guarantee a sleepless night.

To be practical, we decided that we needed more professional
opinions. So we made appointments with Sam's old surgeon, Dr.
Charles White, and with Dr. Ashbrook in Boston. We would see
Dr. White in his office on Long Island on Thursday. He was obviously the perfect choice as a consultant: he knew the whole cast
intimately; David Gaon had worked under him as a resident. On
top of which he was removed from the usual competitiveness by
his specialty, pediatric surgery, and by the fact that he practiced
mostly on the Island. We were especially anxious to hear what he
thought of the continent ileostomy.

Rachel was with us again, this time not on hospital leave, but
duly discharged as of that morning; I'd brought her own coat. We
had immediate, easy rapport with Dr. White; we talked of Sam.
Somehow, in talking to this man who had been instrumental in
saving Sam's life, it seemed permissible to boast: the magna cum
laude, and the job as tennis pro, and last summer at the Supreme
Court as a researcher, and the good law school; even all his girls. I
stopped only when I saw Rachel and Mark exchange raised eyebrows. So we proceeded to Dr. White's endorsement of the Kock
procedure. Not only did he believe in it, but he had successfully
performed several himself. And he told us that he had gone to
watch David Gaon's virtuoso performance several times. "There's
no one better." He added, "If I say so myself!" He smiled; so did
we. It was nice to have a doctor acknowledge his ego needs.

On Friday morning Rachel was bleeding again and had one of
her bad headaches, but we didn't dare postpone the appointment
with Dr. Ashbrook any longer. "So much for the big remission!"
she said to me on the plane. And about the trip, "It's a waste of
time; we know where we're at."

"Daddy has a lot of faith in Dr. Ashbrook's opinion."

"You know what he's going to say." She glanced out the window
at New York tilting away; the ocean looked like a silver-haired
finger wave. "It would be better to get me on the surgical calendar," she said without turning back to me. I didn't answer. I knew
that Dr. Truman had rescheduled their patients' second interview
for May; Rachel was being haunted by that time schedule. Yet,

while I heard her speak of surgery, I did not feel that her decisiveness was real. She was trying out the sound, perhaps.

Daniel was at the airport. Rachel hugged him a long time. It was funny with these two; they didn't know each other very well, because Rachel had only been six when he went off to college. Which sometimes made their communication too damn polite; Rachel found it easier to talk to Ruth. But there was a lot of longing to be close, and on that morning it was important that they were together. I suppose we all knew that it was the decisive day.

What an impressive place Massachusetts General Hospital is! Dr. Ashbrook's office was located in one of the oldest parts of the building, at the end of innumerable corridors, nooks, and turns, the walls adorned with photographs of people from another era in stiff, high collars, with earnest faces, sitting or standing up very straight. I had a sense that the wisdom of the ages was lent to the present in this place. And then Dr. Ashbrook, very accessible, unpretentious, easy to talk to. After examining Rachel, he was certainly the one most positively counseling surgery *now*. Mark and I, our eyes meeting, had both noticed that his glance returned again and again to a certain spot on Rachel's x-ray. He was developing his theory of "activity times duration" for Rachel; he stressed that the operation would turn her into a healthy young woman. "Look at you," he said in his light voice. "You're so pretty, but you look ill. What for? Haven't you been cheated out of enough life?"

The question released her. Suddenly she was discussing with him—the stranger—something none of us had truly verbalized before. "I wouldn't have any doubts except for Paul," she said, looking down on her hands entwined in her lap. Then she looked up, met Dr. Ashbrook's glance. "He's the one I've trusted all my life. And he's brought me through all this time. It's very hard to go against him." She paused, added, "Though I think he'll have to opt for the surgery soon anyhow, but . . . well, it's as if I ought to give him these other few months, that I oughtn't to let him down." Another pause. I opened my mouth to protest, but Dr. Ashbrook raised a hand, stopping me, waiting. And then Rachel burst out, "But I just can't stand to live like this anymore—always saying it's not so bad, never daring to go to a party, have a drink, eat . . ." She bit her lip, fell silent; bright color had flooded into her face. I reached over and took her damp hand; she clutched back tightly.

Dr. Ashbrook said that he understood. He said that it would take courage to tell Paul. "He's become like a father to you," he said. "But we doctors shouldn't treat our own children."

I nodded, agreeing, but then had an odd feeling of shock, of recognition. Such an ordinary statement, such an obvious truism, and I had often said similar things; yet it was only at this moment that I registered what it meant, how important it was. The whole Electra bit: Rachel's love for Paul, her defiance of him, her colossal efforts to make him proud. I felt amazement, almost awe: why hadn't we taken this into consideration; why the need to be told something so much a part of our lives? Oh, I wanted to think about it, speculate, but I also wanted to stay with the conversation and hear what else Dr. Ashbrook had to say. Later, I promised myself; later.

Mark was asking about the continent ileostomy. Dr. Ashbrook said that they did not have much experience with the procedure at Mass General, but that he'd trust to the talent. If Paul recommended it . . . He smiled. "He wouldn't want anything that is bad for you," he said to Rachel. He gave Gaon highest marks. "But the main thing is for you to get rid of this colon." He was staring at the x-ray again. "It's time for you to be well."

Mark and I came together like homing pigeons in the corridor while Rachel was filling Dan in. "There's something in the x-ray that worries him," I said.

"I know."

"Did you know about it before?"

"I wasn't sure. Something Paul said . . ."

I waited.

"A couple of days ago, when Rachel seemed to be so much better, Paul said, 'I don't care what they say, there's no malignancy.' I presumed that he was referring to a dispute about—"

"But you didn't pursue it?" I interrupted.

"No."

We were staring at each other. I knew exactly why Mark had not insisted on clarifying Paul's murky statement; I knew it right then, right there in my stomach, in my gut. I reached out to take Mark's hand.

"He was right that other time when he disagreed with Dr. Baldwin."

"Yes," I agreed. But did not say what had been on my mind ever since Dr. Gaon had explained that the pouch could not be established if there was an involvement of the ileum. I did not say, Well, that's what we're going to sweat out if Rachel goes into surgery. Only then will we really know. Nor did I say that I had never accepted Paul's premise that we'd misunderstood Dr. Baldwin. However, while I didn't say these things, I knew that Mark was as aware of them as I. It wasn't that we were keeping things from each other or even protecting the other's feelings; it was that we were balancing ever so carefully on the crossbar, testing each step to find out how much stress we could endure. Underneath was the abyss; each of us was trying not to fall into it or to push the other. . . .

Rachel came over when Dan went to call his office. "We've changed the plan," she said. The plan had been that Dan was to drive her to the bus—she was going to Providence for the weekend —and us to the airport to fly home. All morning, watching Rachel: the extreme pallor, the obvious pain that caused her to walk stooped, the involuntary gesture of hands flying to clutch her belly when she was hit by spasms; watching and thinking of her getting on that bus caused flushes of terror to course through me. Twice I had already tried to dissuade her from going. She was saying, "Dan had the idea to drive me up to school and that you can fly home from Providence."

"Oh that's marvelous!" Relieved, I turned to Dan, who had finished his call. "Are you sure you can make the time?"

"I've cancelled everything for today."

Then we were sitting in a restaurant; Dan had said that it was known for its good beefburgers. Rachel with her cup of coffee and nothing else. The rest of us ordered the specialty, only to find that it was hard to chew. Suddenly I was angry. "This whole Providence weekend is madness," I burst out. I simply couldn't bear any more fear.

"No, it isn't. I have to see my professors, have to make arrangements." Rachel turned to Mark, said in a quiet voice, "Daddy, could you call Dr. Gaon now? It would help me if I had the date."

In the air again—impossible to believe that it was the same day; I was eons older, I was calmer. We had left Rachel in a cocoon of friends. "Make her eat something," I had begged Len, and he had promised that he would. Outside, the sky was a blank gray; there was nothing to be seen. Now I could open the box I had slammed shut in Dr. Ashbrook's office: his statement that Paul had become a father to Rachel.

Suddenly I remembered something, a snatch of conversation between Paul and Mark, a fragment, unconnected . . . yes, in their living room. Nina had been giving Mark a drink. Paul's face was pale, his voice loud. "I'm just a stand-in for you," he said. "It's you she's angry at." I strained for more: what was the context? But nothing appeared—only my face reflected in the window.

So Paul had understood. Or only partly understood? Rachel's part, not his own, not his loss of objectivity? Had there been a breakdown in professional judgment? Had he allowed Rachel to walk around with a time bomb ticking away? Who could judge? Not I with all my fine psychological jargon and my nice theoretical knowledge. And even if I *knew*, could I feel it where it might count? Count for what? What difference would it make whether I loved or hated Paul? Perhaps no one had made a mistake. Only nature. And perhaps no one could have made the decision before today. Certainly no one except Rachel. It had had to ripen. I pictured the disease as a horrid fruit on a tree that still bore tender yellow blossoms.

"It's just as well that there's another exacerbation," Mark said, breaking into my thoughts. "At least it removes my last doubt." Then he told me that Dr. Gaon had said on the telephone that he had run into Paul the previous evening. "Paul told him that Rachel would be having the surgery forthwith." Paul had asked Gaon to put Rachel on the surgical calendar.

CHAPTER 14

ALSO FROM RACHEL'S POEM:
AT LAST, THE FOREST A CATHEDRAL

Some quest,
*   some newly opened, closed mind brought me here.*
But it is cold in and out among these trees.

Rachel came back from Providence on February 15; I took her straight to Dr. Freund's office from the airport. She was scheduled to go into Mt. Sinai Hospital on the twenty-sixth. Was she having enough time to prepare herself? And had the daily sessions with Dr. Freund helped her to make the decision? I had no idea.

In the meantime, we had these ten days. Endless days that succeeded one another too fast. The night terrors: the spot on the x-ray, the exacerbation—dear God, please, not now, not when it is already decided. Just let her be able to get the pouch; don't let anything blow. I had a recurring dream in which Rachel wandered, lost, in a milky landscape. Just that; she was a little girl in the dream, holding her belly. And while nothing happened, I knew that she had a megacolon and was somewhere far from help. I'd wake, my throat parched, and the dream terror would deepen as I thought, What if she hadn't been at Lenox Hill Hospital that time of the incipient megacolon? And how could we have permitted her to go back to school after that? And all the "what if's" piling into my mind, sleep flown. I'd hear the rustle of Mark's Gelusil paper and the clink of his water glass, and even when he slept, his moans and cries. We were aware of each other all night long, though we seldom talked; sometimes we held hands. And outside our door, Rachel's steps and the small click of her light switch at every hour, or a book falling down. And the ticking of the bomb.

In the mornings we met bleary-eyed. The bright spots came unexpectedly. Yes, the laughs. A girl with whom Dr. Gaon had put Rachel in touch, who had had the continent ileostomy established the previous summer, was "crazy about it!"

"She sounds so . . . so free, so blithe," Rachel reported. "Mom, you should have heard her. Nothing is a problem; she bubbles; she says that she doesn't know why she waited so long, that it's a new world. And that she used to be so sick! 'My stoma is so small; hell, on special occasions I just wear a Band-Aid over it!' she said." Rachel giggled. "And she says that when she goes to classes, she just sticks her catheter into her knee socks or into the hip pocket of her jeans." Rachel snapped her fingers. "Like: no sweat!" All that day, Rachel went around smiling. So did Mark and I. To think that there could be carefreeness! A girl could go to college without worry and wear a Band-Aid for special occasions.

A more sober evaluation came from a woman in her late thirties. But she was also very positive. "Though of course," Rachel said to us, "she was already married and had had her kids before all this happened. And she was never on any immunosuppressive agents, so her chromosomes didn't get fucked up." The chromosomes, the drugs she had been taking over the long years, the messed-up chemical system—these were Rachel's nightmare worries. She also talked about responsibility. How much of the disease had she brought upon herself? And wasn't Paul's reluctance to opt for the surgery a sign that he hadn't considered her really sick? Yet she knew that she couldn't go on; ergo: it must be her fault. What force inside of her was getting in the way of her wish to be creative, to live, to be well?

Appalled, impatient, I argued.

"I hope she's working on this with Dr. Freund," I said to Mark. "I just can't bear that on top of everything else, she's beating herself with this nonsense."

"It's not nonsense. Those are legitimate thoughts she has to test."

"I know, I know. I just hate it so. But you're right, she has to work through it so that she can discard those guilts once and for all." Then thought ironically, The way we have disposed of our guilt? Oh, if only it didn't take forever to explore such matters; I wished I could just pooh-pooh the whole thing away, joke her out of it, kiss it away the way I had kissed away the little scratches of her babyhood. But of course, it was one more thing with which I could not help. Out loud I said, "Just the same, it ought to be a comfort to her to know that we're solidly in her corner."

"You mean in the fight of Rachel versus Rachel? In which corner?"

"In the 'you didn't bring this upon yourself' corner."

"Are we?"

"Come on, Mark," I said angrily. "You know that we don't believe that Rachel is responsible for any of this. Why, your work with the Foundation should have taught you that—the whole direction of all the doctors. None of them consider ulcerative colitis a psychogenic disease."

"No. But we've been plenty upset many times—when she would not take care of herself, when she insisted on going to school though she was sick as a dog, when she didn't eat properly, and the time she had to go to Israel . . ."

"And denying the pain," I added.

"See?"

I nodded. Oh, God, if we had such thoughts, how much more cruelly they must plague Rachel. And was I being supportive enough? Perhaps my impatience, my reluctance to have her discuss it with me had signified my own uncertainty? When, *really*, I had none. Or was I protesting just a little too much? She wasn't the only one who had a tendency to deny. . . .

Somehow, we got through the days until that Saturday. How terrible was my efficiency—I knew exactly what to pack: her pillow, her heating pad, the plants that thrived best under hospital fluorescent lamps, and the Kelly green towels. We were there with her in Admissions: Mark and Sam and I. I would not cry when they put the plastic I.D. around her wrist; it was such an incredible repetition. I looked once into Sam's closed, white face; it was as if he did not live behind those features. Then I tried not to glance at him again. He stayed close to Rachel, physically in reach.

Her room was large, looking out over the park. We got there with her things before Rachel, who had to go through an admissions procedure of having a chest x-ray and blood tests taken. It appeared to us that she preferred to go along with the aide without her retinue. So I unpacked and then, maniacally, washed the soot off the windowpanes. I kept showing Mark the black paper towels, saying, "Look at that. Can you imagine, can you imagine how filthy . . . " And even after Rachel came in, I was still full of conversation about the dirty windows. And where shall I put this poster? "Here? It will hide the scratches on the closet door. Okay?" Rachel said fine, that would be fine. But took the roll that contained the image of the little cat hanging tough on the chinning bar out of my hand. She smoothed it and then Scotch-Taped it to the bathroom door herself.

It seemed to me that by the next morning Rachel was in another world from us. Yes, this was different from being sick at Lenox Hill; this was coming into an environemnt geared to convert from illness to health. Norma Berliner said so. She would be Rachel's morning nurse; she was bubbling and warm. I listened to her as she explained that everyone on the team was excited about the Kock procedure, everyone was specially trained, everyone was positive. (What did they do with the mavericks, I wondered? With the nurse or resident who didn't share the enthusiasm? Did they deport them, whoosh off the seventh floor?) Norma also told me that everyone was in love with Dr. Gaon and that Rachel had already had a visit from Arthur, who was three weeks postop, and that she could see Joan later. "Joan was done Wednesday," she said. Overwhelmed after this encounter, but also impressed, I entered Rachel's room. "Wow, she's something!"

Rachel laughed.

"But you know, there is no doubt that this is a good setup for the patient."

"Why?"

"The positive atmosphere, everyone pulling together . . ."

"Oh, Mom, you're romanticizing. I think it's just Norma. The floor nurses do not seem terribly involved. And as for Arthur, well, since Norma has already told me his life history, I just hope that she didn't tell him mine."

"Well, luckily she doesn't know all your dark secrets," I answered, peeved that Rachel had burst my bubble. I'd felt so good there for a moment.

"I got the timetable," Rachel said, becoming a little more animated. "This really nice surgical resident was in. But, my luck, he's going off the service on the first. But *he's* really involved; he says that he admires all the 'pouchies,' that it takes a lot of courage to opt for something so new. Anyhow, he gave me the countdown. The operation is on Friday. Tomorrow they're starting me on the blood transfusions—"

"Why? Because you're so anemic?"

"I didn't ask. I assume that I am. And that they want me in the best possible shape for the O.R." Suddenly she stopped, her eyes wide. I put my arms around her and we sat quietly. After a while I wondered what it was that made me so profoundly sad just at that moment, and then knew. Not just that she couldn't say she was scared. No, that Rachel said that she hadn't asked why she was to have the blood transfusions.

Later, returning from an errand, I found her bed empty, a note propped against the pillow. *"Have gone to see Joan. Come on up, her nurse says it's okay."* I shook my head, no, I didn't want to go. I sat down, picked up one of Rachel's books, started to read. But it was impossible to concentrate. First of all, who could stand this stuff? *Dying in America.* And then the thoughts—the recoil at the idea of seeing this Joan, four days postop. No, please, not yet. And only then took in the information that the date was set for next Friday. So soon. When the telephone rang, it was Rachel. "Why don't you come up? Joan says she'd like to meet you; she is fantastic."

"Tomorrow, perhaps," I said weakly. "It's too early to impose."

"She says nonsense. Tell Dad to come too."

Mark walking in just then, catching the drift, shook his head violently. After I'd hung up, he said, "Dear God, not that too."

But then later in the afternoon we got dragged upstairs after all. I felt that we were being tested. If we could not take the sight of this strange girl, how would we react to her? Oh I recognized the syndrome; Rachel wouldn't spare us any more than Sam had.

Joan was connected to several bottles which converged into an I.V. in her forearm. She was a little girl, making not much of a bulge under the sheet; her face had an expression of listening inward. I admired her flowers, her plants, and the collection of get-well cards and ribbons that surrounded the bed. She kept saying, "It's just my back that is so bad." The nurse, Carla, promised that the morphine would work soon, then she would be more comfortable. Carla and Rachel talked. Joan was really doing splendidly; her bladder catheter was already out and she was urinating on her own. But much more remarkably, "They took out the N.G. tube this morning already." Turning to me, Carla explained,

"That is really unusually fast. As a rule, they keep the pouchies on the stomach pump for at least a week." Joan was smiling proudly.

"Arthur's was in for two weeks," Rachel contributed.

"And Bonnie's—you'll meet her tomorrow. She's coming for her posthospital checkup and will visit Joan. I'll send her down to see you," Carla promised Rachel. "Anyhow, Bonnie had some trouble . . ."

Please, please, I thought, don't tell us. I glanced at Mark, who hadn't said a word. Not like me. Babbling along with the girls. Oh, yes, the hospital gowns were much more practical than nightgowns, but it was better for the morale to get into something pretty. "That's why I did Joan's hair with dry shampoo," Carla said. Joan nodded, fingered her hair; her eyes weren't focusing quite right. At last Mark said heartily, "I think we should let Joan get some rest now!" We all nodded, though Joan was already asleep. But then she roused herself and said politely that she was sorry that we had missed her mother. "But she had to go back to Washington." We made awkward farewells.

In the elevator with Rachel, I was furious at her, then melted with regret and pity and guilt as she said, "See, they don't let you be uncomfortable for long."

In the next few days Arthur became a part of our life. He was always in Rachel's room; he came from San Francisco, and he was lonesome. Some of his stories made me wince. He had this awful male night nurse who'd always gone to sleep, so it had fallen to Arthur to keep the watch and wake the guy to do his hourly irrigation. With the result that now, allowed to sleep three hours at a stretch, Arthur couldn't sleep. He had deep dark circles under his eyes. He warned Rachel to be very tough with her nurses. "Just throw them out if they're not good." We nodded obediently.

Arthur also had strong opinions on diet. He spoke eloquently about the foods that couldn't agree with pouchies, "Regardless what Gaon might say!" and about others which, while on the forbidden list, were perfectly harmless. On and on; also on the subject of never trusting people to understand about being sick if they hadn't experienced it for themselves. "I never told anyone, not even my girlfriend."

Sometimes Rachel would make signs of exasperation behind his back; we would have liked to be alone more, but didn't have the heart to keep him out. So we would wait until the alarm clock he carried in the pocket of his robe went off, signifying that he had to get back to his room to empty or irrigate. And anyhow, perhaps it was just as well, because we had an even harder time when we were alone; talk didn't flow, it sprang up painfully, in snatches. And almost every subject was hot; we'd drop it quickly, tongues burned. As about the blood in its plastic sack. Slowly, it dripped into Rachel's vein. From the minute I had come in the morning and seen it, it had scared and depressed me. When Arthur finally left, I pointed to it, said, "It makes it so damn official."

We both stared at the dark bag.

Then, abruptly, Rachel asked, "Is Paul mad at me?"

"Heavens, of course not!" I protested quickly. "I told you, he's been terribly busy. Dad spoke to him last night."

"It's just so strange without him."

"I know." For me too. The internist now on the case was a stranger, though I was bending over backward trying to like him. There was probably nothing wrong with him except that he wasn't Paul. It occurred to me at that moment that we had discussed the fact that Paul wouldn't attend Rachel if she went to Mt. Sinai for the surgery only in terms of what it would mean to her health. There had been no question that between Dr. Gaon and this gastroenterologist recommended by Paul she would be in good hands. We hadn't spoken of how it would affect Paul. Had it been an emotional matter that had kept him from visiting her? In spite of my quick denial, I had been wondering myself.

As far as I knew, Paul's decision to switch from Mt. Sinai to Lenox Hill had been a gradual process. For a while he had used both hospitals. If I had thought of it at all, I must have assumed that this had become impractical. Or perhaps the chances of advancement were more favorable at Lenox Hill. But now I wondered, had there been other factors? Politics, maybe? Was it painful for Paul to walk into Mt. Sinai, which had been home base for him those many years? Or had he really been too busy?

However, that afternoon, coming downstairs on my way to feed the monster parking meter, I ran into him. He was on his way to see Rachel, but it was slow going; he kept meeting people who greeted him enthusiastically. Whatever had prompted his switch to another hospital, it wasn't that he had no friends at this one. Just the same, he was under strain, perspiration on his forehead, a special huskiness in his voice. When we walked into Rachel's room, I felt compelled to clown, to sing out a drumroll, in order to cut through the high emotion.

A couple of minutes later I was back outside in the corridor. From what had I fled? From witnessing what tragedy? Or perhaps it was I who was making all this drama? I who projected it onto the others? But I thought not. There had been the moment when Rachel had caught sight of Paul and her face had broken into angular shards. Relief and grief and anger? Oh, a lot of emotions, but to verbalize them was a luxury we couldn't afford. This "end of the road" image was dangerous to the concept that we were at the start of a journey into health. And then I was suddenly furious —who needed all this? It might have been so much easier if there had been consensus among the doctors, if the decision making hadn't been put on Rachel. Goddamnit, why should she have the burden of wondering yet whether Paul was mad at her?

The feeling of happiness and relief I had experienced when I had seen him come swinging through the revolving doors was gone; dry-eyed, I reentered the room. They were laughing. Rachel was regaling Paul with hospital gossip, of which she had already accumulated a considerable amount. After a while a couple of nurses stopped in, glad to see Paul; everyone had a good time. I watched and felt as if I had wandered into an alien world, a world where only I dwelt. But after Paul had left, Rachel cried. And then got mad. "Why the hell should it matter so much what he thinks?" she asked, and rubbed the tears off her cheeks.

"Did he say anything to upset you?"

"No. He was lovely." She tried to grin. "Not even one joke."

"It's hard on him too." Oh, God, listen to me. . . .

"Cut it out, Mom," Rachel said sharply.

There followed a couple of days during which Rachel was without the intravenous—"off the leash," as she put it. The blood transfusions had actually put pink into her cheeks; she was beautiful with her large golden eyes, long hair, and a quality that I could not quite define. Perhaps it was a sort of peace that had wrapped itself around her as she settled into the routine of the surgical preparation. To be committed and not to have to make new decisions; to be cared for and not to carry responsibility for the daily management.

The ulcerative colitis was in its final flare; Rachel was bleeding and had pain—"Lest I forget what this is all about!" she said. I was sure it was a tremendous relief to be able to give in and take the painkiller the nurse brought her, not to have to worry about whether she could afford to be groggy or if she must stay alert for chemistry. I even noted that she wasn't touching the row of books on death and dying that lined the windowsill and made her visitors uneasy; she was reading a novel. Yes, acceptance. For me too. If not for the fear, we might have enjoyed the sluttishness of watching soap operas, of having laid down the reins; but there was the fear. Sharp and cold and many-faceted, it lay in my stomach, a horrible diamond. Rachel didn't verbalize hers. Only sometimes, her eyes would suddenly widen and she would stop in the middle of whatever she was saying. . . .

I think maybe more than anyone else, Sam was good for her. She liked it if he sat there, reading a law book, just being with her. They didn't have the intense talks they had had at the time when Rachel first considered the surgery on a conscious level. Then she had wanted to question him endlessly, compulsively, for hours at a clip. It had bewildered all of us. "How could she know so little about it?" Sam asked. "I mean, living under one roof . . ." It came up between Rachel and myself now, and I said, "It seems strange you should have been so inattentive to Sam's emotional problems, so insensitive to the climate in which he lives. But I suppose you blocked out everything concerning an ileostomy."

Rachel shook her head, no. "No, I don't think so; I don't think I blocked out anything; but when I asked Sam all those questions, I just had to hear what lay between his answers and the truth I had observed."

Her reply shocked me. I sat silently, mulling it over. Then Rachel added, "It wasn't to entrap Sam . . . just, well, wanting to know how everything seemed to him. Truth being relative. The only truth we have is what we think we feel; it was comforting to see that there is protective coloring."

"I don't think that I understand."

She smiled a little. "Okay, it's a little hazy to me too—I mean, now that it has passed. But it seemed very important then to measure whether one has to know everything. And if one doesn't, if that blinds one to all the vital issues. Sam's answers reassured me. But of course, I have no guarantee that I'll do as well as he."

"You'll do fantastically."

"You are no help with your unbridled prejudice." She laughed.

Another comfort came from the wholehearted support of her friends. Olivia and Douglas Bradshaw, the Trumans, Len and all the kids who'd gone through these terrible times with her. Though Len's approval seemed to rub her wrong. "He's been pushing too damn hard for it," she complained. "And it isn't he who's going to be carved up." I didn't answer that one. It would have been silly; she must have known whatever I might have said. And somehow I could understand this crazy resentment against the friend who'd been so good to her; there was too damned much indebtedness. She illustrated it with an incident that had taken place during her time at school between the first and second stays at Lenox Hill when Len had constantly checked up on her. "God, I needed so much to be alone, but he was always dropping by or telephoning." And then one night when she was in very bad pain they had been on the telephone and she kept telling him that she'd be all right, not to come over, that she had taken Talwin and that as soon as it worked, she'd do some chemistry.

As she told me about it, Rachel sat up in bed, pushed the hair out of her face, said, "And Mom, you know how I couldn't eat at the time, so the Talwin really hit me. Anyhow, I guess I fell asleep, though Len, of course, says I passed out. I'd been sitting on the floor; the telephone and my books were on the bed. But next thing I knew I was in bed and it was early morning and Len was sitting at my desk, working." She paused, thought, added, "I know it's not fair, but it still makes me furious! I mean, yes, he got scared when I fell asleep without hanging up the phone, and he came over. Then Linda and he got me into bed, and then he didn't want to leave me alone. But just the same . . ." Voice rising: "It's high-handed, isn't it? I hate it."

I said that I understood, but that she was wrong, of course. "Len saw what was driving all of us crazy, this denial of yours, making nothing of the pain. And that was already after the megacolon; you were playing with fire, and that whole return to school was madness."

She answered impatiently. "Yes, yes, I know that. But don't you see, to wake up and find that I was not alone, it was an invasion too. He was forcing his will, his judgment on me. Even if he was right. And it so happens, when things really went wrong, I made all the right moves; I called Paul and—"

I interrupted, "You were lucky. That Paul was in, that the Bradshaws were able to come. But Len was there too. If Livvie and Doug hadn't been able to make it in that weather, he would have gotten you to a hospital."

"That's true." She was tired, leaned back; I realized that recalling these nightmare incidents had exhausted her. I also realized that Len would always be guilty of his good deed. Weird, the human heart.

The countdown: one day on a soft diet, one on liquids, and then nothing *per os*. And endless flushing of the intestines. Disagreeable, sometimes painful, sad. That was when Mark cheered us no end with his "Don't think of it as losing a colon; think of it as gaining a pouch!" We laughed inordinately.

Mark and I went home on the evening before the surgery, leaving Rachel with Sam and Jack. Jack had brought a second Megillah scroll along, so Sam perched on the bed next to Rachel and they followed Jack's chanting of the ancient text. At each mention of the villainous Haman it is customary to whir a *gregor*, a noise-maker; but it seemed an inappropriate thing to do in a hospital, so instead they pounded softly on the tray table and against the metal railing of the bed. The two tall young men in their *yarmulkes* and Rachel in her prettiest nightgown, it was very meaningful to all of them; they had been friends almost all their lives. And of course for Jack, who is very religious, it was also a fulfillment of the command to read the Megillah to a sick person—a *mitzvah*. But for Sam and Rachel it was Tradition with orchestration from the Fiddler. Except with more fervor than irony, because ritual is wonderfully comforting in the bad moments of life. The Megillah had been read by their grandfathers and would be read by their children. Making the assumption that the chain would not be broken.

After the boys had left, Rachel washed her hair, and then she wrote a long letter to Paul. I guess it said all the things she hadn't been able to say—that she thanked him, that he was a part of her life, that she hoped that he would be in her future. As her friend.

We got back to the seventh floor at six A.M. Sam was already sitting on the bench by the elevator. "They are shaving Rachel," he said.

"Did you get home at all?" I asked.

"Sure. I had plenty of sleep."

"We did too."

We waited until the nurse motioned us in. Outside, it was beginning to get light. It was raining. A forgotten tear lay in the hollow under Rachel's eye; I kissed it away. Then babbled—it was such a relief that it was no longer part of prepping for surgery to insert all the tubes and catheters while the patient is awake. She'd have none of this disagreeable stuff, would just go to sleep . . . Rachel's absent look finally shut me up. Then we just stood around, Mark walked over, bent down, and kissed her; Sam held her hand. Nurses wandered in and out; the surgical resident came by, said, "See you soon, Rachel," and left again. She told us that the anesthetist had seen her the previous evening; yes, he seemed nice. "Good thing it isn't cold outside. Can you imagine if all this rain were snow? We wouldn't have made it," I said.

Rachel smiled. Like: so? The machinery would have worked without us too. The assembly line, moving parts from belt to belt. And there was the orderly with the stretcher; he was very tall and quite old. And jovial. I don't know what all we said in the hall. I just remember Rachel's crooked smile and that she told us to keep busy, that she'd be occupied for a while. But Mark said that she cried and cautioned us not to suffer like this. We also said, "I love you" all around. Then I had the weird feeling that I was seeing the scene from her perspective—flat on my back, the I.V. bottles swaying above me, the corridor walls rushing by, seeming to tilt inward to make a tent over me. And the attendant calling, "Hold the elevator!"

Epilogue I

Brown University
Providence, R.I.
June 30, 1977

Dear Mom and Dad,

I don't think we communicated very well just now. In fact, it was a distinctly behind-the-looking-glass conversation. You, Dad, saying "Well, if you don't have time . . ." in a hurt voice, and Mom getting antsy to get off the phone.

But perhaps I can explain it in writing. It's just that it took such time and effort to settle back here; I really wasn't sure that I'd be able to do it—all the kids in the midst of finals and the general "end of the year, thank God it's over" hysteria. And me so out of it, suddenly thinking words like: alienation. But they are gone now, and the campus is lovely, empty, serene; life is slow-paced. I need this time to get my head together before school starts again in the fall, and I am glad that it is deserted and that I am alone; I don't think I could deal with my well-intentioned but overly concerned friends at this point.

So I've plunged myself back into the academics. I've finished up the Am Civ and my Soc and gotten A's in both. Doug's giving me an A in the research project too, but I'm still struggling with Reli Stu. I'll have to redo the paper entirely if I want to shoot for an A. It's not that it doesn't interest me anymore; it's just difficult to pick up after this long time. Or perhaps it's a bad moment in my life to deal with abstractions —with one *more* abstraction, in any case. Though, I guess, I will give it another try.

More important than that, I must finish up my interviews. I was feeling very nervous about returning to them; I wondered whether I would be able to maintain my objectivity after everything that has happened to me recently. But it went okay; I settled back into it with no difficulty. A number of the patients I saw knew that I'd been ill—they had inquired when they didn't see me for this long time—which, somehow, did not hurt at all. In any case, we have lost only one patient. He died in March already, but Adam didn't want to tell me because I was only a few days postop at the time.

Anyhow, all this is pretty long-winded just to repeat that I won't be coming home for the Fourth of July weekend. And as you can see, it's not really the work as much as the fact that I don't want to come home right now, don't want to lie in the sun or look at the ocean or even play tennis. I seem to feel that I'm in the middle of something more imperative—my first tentative steps toward "getting on with it." Do you know what I mean?

I also told you on the telephone that I've written this poem. Well, I've decided to send it to you. In fact, if you can use it for the book, Mom, help yourself. One thing is sure: until it poured out of me, I didn't fully comprehend that I had been unable, rather than unwilling, to accept the danger in which I had been. Perhaps that is the single most difficult thing to deal with when one is ill—this concept of *knowing*; knowing the full peril, knowing the inner fury, recognizing the awful mixture of longing, submission, and sexuality with which a person responds to the nearness of death.

Please let me know what you think. And please understand.

Love,
Rachel

AT LAST, THE FOREST A CATHEDRAL
by

Rachel Bergman

The child is lost.
Deep in this jungle of thoughts,
tangled emotions,
web of fear,
forest of words . . .
a thicket of unasked questions.
The chain saws have started their rasp . . .

how to still their roar?
Or should I even try?

Some quest, some newly opened, closed mind brought me here.
But it is cold in and out of these trees,
and the child got lost
chasing after phantom dreams of freedom,
not isolation.
Singing ancient songs of courage, of victory,
dreaming poetry of unscaled heights . . . beyond this clearing.
Oh, no, this can not be.
Don't push, girl, don't push.

The new God, the old one failed, you know.
Just a man, a doctor.
A new chance, a better way.
Orderly,
trees planted in a row.
But what has this to do with me?
Not me, no, never.
O power!
It is too convincing . . .
Soul,
are you prepared to carry my devastated carcass?

Only twenty, really thirty, maybe more.
But lonely and longing.
Just twenty, and too many needs.
Yearning, but afraid
to fly, to soar, maybe to crash.
Hide me, forest! Cover me, thicket . . .
Or I face what I know not of.
Flesh, heir to pain,
I hate you.

Why can't I turn it off?
Try! It has to work.
No? Damn saws—they reduced my cover to stumps.
Menacing nakedness,
stripped, sliced apart.
Yet still trees, the same but different.

Altered status.
Go away, it is too personal now.
Don't you know?
She can not find her way.
The landscape has changed.

Okay, gamble for life. No, I mean gamble for a new life.
But do it now.
Consensus, Gods! Please, you are tearing me apart.
Human, fallible, yessiree!
GODS!
The lost child has agreed.
Hold her hand,
guide her along these untrod jungle paths.
But hurry, her pioneer daring might not last.

Talking jags—sadistic?
Why not?
Bleed with me, hurt.
That feels so good.
To be kissed and hugged.
Love me, please! Here, now.
The forest will hide us . . .
   boughs as canopy, mossy bed,
   underbrush a flimsy cover for rocking bodies.
OVERWHELMED!
By pleasure, by pain.

Damn routine, thermometer, pulse, pitcher.
It will get worse.
GONE, the safety of my green hiding place.
But I have new escape—
   it comes in pills and needles.
Good morning, God. A fun agenda . . . prepping for surgery:
   sterilize the gut
   vomit the thoughts
Oh, never hostile!
Indignities are on the way out.

So the morning of the day is here.
Enter players!

Any problems?
No, not a one. Except to play the farewell scene.
Try it one day,
full of happy pills and the pressure of terror.
So long, do something nice.
I shall be busy for a while.

Separate.
Alone.
The same but different.
There is freedom in possessing no thing, you know.
And fear in limitless possibilities . . .
But all this later. Have to concentrate on healing.

Raped body;
some new devices for your pleasure—
bottles, tubes, machines.
And the memory of the recovery room agony fading
*   but forever part of me now.*
Back from the dead . . .
heightened awareness.
Do not look now, but . . .
it is all over. It is just beginning.

Morphine euphoria,
relief.
But really now, God, enough!
You have run out of all the time I shall give you.
The child's fury is growing, an awesome thing.
She is impatient,
intolerant of her incomplete life.

Back from the nothing.
There is something to lose again.
Careful, you different, same being . . .
beyond the red,
*   beyond the blood and pain*
It is blue!
Will it last?
This second long feeling of
BEING ALIVE.

Exaltation
  after tortured days.
Sublime beauty
  in easing pain.
So my death is a lie.
I will live a lifetime.
Not in a year, day, or moment.
In a lifetime.

Which makes it my turn, God.
Despairing to find self-confidence,
Understand! What I am I shall always be.
Ambivalent me; wants her day too.
To love, to hate,
to
CRUSH
CRACK
BANG
All you guys together.
Yet preserve the love, the safety?
Punish the impotence.

Back from that gray zone at twenty.
In search of vitality,
with time to dream, to be inspired.
Trembling with desire
  to be serious about life.
Child, use your time!
Sun rays piercing treetops.
At last, the forest a cathedral,
though far off, the crash of dying giants.
And I am dying still.
So, LIVE! Grow.

In the year of my rebirth ...
this year
of deep despair,
consuming rage,
and stay of execution ...
I touched tongues with death.

Epilogue II

by   Rachel Bergman

THANKSGIVING 1977

Since the poem was written, almost six months ago, much has happened. To attempt to write a postscript to my mother's skillful weaving of time and incident is hard. What additional perspective can I offer; what insight will complete my story with realism and honesty? Or perhaps I only want to offer one more undisguised confidence, one more unabashed, unflattering exposure of my inner world . . . my reaction now, at twenty-one, when I look back at what has been. And when I look ahead at what is still to come.

There have been so many new and big adjustments to be struggled with, and new disappointments with which I must deal: next month I will again be leaving school, interrupting my life again, to go back to Mt. Sinai Hospital for additional surgery: a revision, they call it. Because the valve that is to keep the pouch continent has unraveled and must be rebuilt and repositioned. The need for this surgery, to have to go back to the hospital, to put myself under someone else's control again, to be hooked up once more to all sorts of tubes, I.V.s, bedside bags, and most of all, to have pain again when I finally know the joy of waking in the morning to a body which does not hurt . . . to call that a major disappointment is a ridiculous understatement.

So I look back to the moment when the poem was written. It was in a fantastic mood of relief. Relief to be back in life—to be alive—to have a full and unrestricted future to look forward to. It is a poem of hope and joy and of expectation. But it also deals with the rage and despair and the fear which were as truly devastating as the sense of rebirth is exhilarating.

There has been much in these months which has demanded considerable adaptation from me; I have been forced to stand naked before myself, exposed and vulnerable, in the hope that doing so would allow me to understand what it is to be and to feel human, to accept myself within the context of my entire spectrum of feelings. My identity has been threatened, both profoundly and minutely. I am not what I always was in the past, because I no longer experience—and thus fit into—my old world in quite the same way as I did before. Yet I am the same person. A big dilemma: the same yet different. How to relate to the world now? And how to integrate the nightmares of these past years into the totality of my life, when, as yet, they represent the majority of my years. These are just a few of the current life problems—trying to find out where my real self is, and who it is, in the midst of all this confusion. And it seems as if I presently have so many selves—confused ones, lost ones, blind ones—how to discover the real one? Perhaps, among the many, I will one day birth a triumphant one.

Maybe the single greatest problem that exists is my overwhelming weariness right now. It is so pervasive that it leaves me absolutely afraid to have to feel anything more; I am psychically numb, as it were. And this stasis forms a barrier to the kind of living and feeling I need for creativity, autonomy, self-actualization. And self-understanding. In other words, less pretentiously: it keeps me from getting on with it. . . .

So what am I trying to say? Do I regret my decision? Do I think that it was wrong? I wish I could answer unequivocally that I don't—not for a moment—ever. But that would be ignoring the continuing agony of the questioning. That would deny depressions and doubts. And yet I know that "I will live a lifetime . . ." now, fully and productively, a healthy woman. Just as soon as I stop being so weary. I guess what I am saying is that the experience does not end with hospital discharge. A great deal of work is required—and not only from the surgeon—in attempting to transform a body that has sustained twelve years of illness and massive drug infusion into a normal, healthy, vibrant individual.

I suppose I was naive. Because I did not expect this. I thought that things would fall in line more quickly and easily. One kiss from the prince . . . I did not expect to still have to struggle so desperately hard.

Maybe, during the upcoming hospitalization, we can find a poster of a donkey standing patiently in the desert. The caption to counsel: Patience, Jackass, *Patience*.

AUTHOR'S NOTE

A bibliography of articles on ileitis and colitis is available at the
    National Foundation for Ileitis and Colitis, Inc.
    295 Madison Avenue, New York, New York 10017
    Telephone: (212) 685-3440.
Staff and volunteers will be glad to assist anyone interested in obtaining information; pamphlets discussing various aspects of inflammatory bowel diseases and other educational material will be sent upon request.